Arthroplasty Around the Wrist: CMC, Radiocarpal, DRUJ

Editor

MARWAN A. WEHBÉ

HAND CLINICS

www.hand.theclinics.com

Consulting Editor
KEVIN C. CHUNG

February 2013 • Volume 29 • Number 1

ELSEVIER

1600 John F. Kennedy Blvd. • Suite 1800 • Philadelphia, Pennsylvania 19103

http://www.theclinics.com

HAND CLINICS Volume 29, Number 1
February 2013 ISSN 0749-0712, ISBN-13: 978-1-4557-7096-0

Editor: David Parsons

Hand Clinics (ISSN 0749-0712) is published quarterly by Elsevier Inc., 360 Park Avenue South, New York, NY 10010-1710. Months of publication are February, May, August, and November. Business and Editorial Offices: 1600 John F. Kennedy Blvd., Ste. 1800, Philadelphia, PA 19103-2899. Customer Service Office: 3251 Riverport Lane, Maryland Heights, MO 63043. Periodicals postage paid at New York, NY and at additional mailing offices. Subscription price is $368.00 per year (domestic individuals), $583.00 per year (domestic institutions), $184.00 per year (domestic students/residents), $420.00 per year (Canadian individuals), $666.00 per year (Canadian institutions), $500.00 per year (international individuals), $666.00 per year (international institutions), and $243.00 per year (international and Canadian students/residents). Foreign air speed delivery is included in all *Clinics* subscription prices. All prices are subject to change without notice. **POSTMASTER:** Send address changes to *Hand Clinics*, Elsevier Health Sciences Division, Subscription Customer Service, 3251 Riverport Lane, Maryland Heights, MO 63043. Customer Service (orders, claims, online, change of address): Elsevier Health Sciences Division, Subscription Customer Service, 3251 Riverport Lane, Maryland Heights, MO 63043. Tel: 1-800-654-2452 (U.S. and Canada); 314-447-8871 (outside U.S. and Canada). Fax: 314-447-8029. E-mail: journalscustomerservice-usa@elsevier.com (for print support); journalsonlinesupport-usa@elsevier.com (for online support).

Reprints. For copies of 100 or more of articles in this publication, please contact the Commercial Reprints Department, Elsevier Inc., 360 Park Avenue South, New York, New York 10010-1710. Tel.: 212-633-3812; Fax: 212-462-1935; E-mail: reprints@elsevier.com.

Hand Clinics is covered in *MEDLINE/PubMed (Index Medicus), Current Contents/Clinical Medicine, EMBASE/Excerpta Medica,* and *ISI/BIOMED.*

Printed and bound by CPI Group (UK) Ltd, Croydon, CR0 4YY

Transferred to digital print 2012

Contributors

CONSULTING EDITOR

KEVIN C. CHUNG, MD
Charles B.G. de Nancrede Professor of
Surgery, Section of Plastic Surgery,
Department of Surgery, Assistant Dean for
Faculty Affairs, Associate Director of Global
REACH, University of Michigan Medical
School, The University of Michigan Health
System, Ann Arbor, Michigan

GUEST EDITOR

MARWAN A. WEHBÉ, MD
Medical Director, Pennsylvania Hand Center,
Bryn Mawr, Pennsylvania; Professor
Orthopaedic and Hand Surgery, Jefferson
Medical College, Philadelphia, Pennsylvania

AUTHORS

BRIAN D. ADAMS, MD
Professor of Orthopedic Surgery, Chief of
Hand Surgery and Director of Hand Surgery
Fellowship, Orthopedic Surgery, University of
Iowa, Iowa City, Iowa

RICHARD A. BERGER, MD, PhD
Professor, Orthopedic Surgery and Anatomy,
Chair, Division of Hand Surgery, Orthopedic
Surgery, Mayo Clinic, Rochester, Minnesota

RICHARD I. BURTON, MD
Professor, Department of Orthopaedics,
Senior Associate Dean for Academic Affairs,
School of Medicine and Dentistry, University of
Rochester Medical Center, Rochester,
New York

RITA M. CICCARELLO, RN
Clinical Assistant, Pennsylvania Hand Center,
Bryn Mawr, Pennysylvania

CARLA A. CROSBY, PT, CHT
Hand Therapy Department, Pennsylvania Hand
Center, Bryn Mawr, Pennsylvania

JOHN C. ELFAR, MD
Assistant Professor, Department of
Orthopaedics, School of Medicine and
Dentistry, University of Rochester Medical
Center, Rochester, New York

MARC GARCIA-ELIAS, MD, PhD
Institut Kaplan for Surgery of the Hand and
Upper Extremity, Barcelona, Spain

MARIE-LYNE GRENIER, MSc, OTR/L
Hand Therapy Department, Pennsylvania Hand
Center, Bryn Mawr, Pennsylvania

ALBERTO L. LLUCH, MD, PhD
Institut Kaplan for Surgery of the Hand and
Upper Extremity, Barcelona, Spain

ALEX B. LLUCH, MD
Institut Kaplan for Surgery of the Hand and
Upper Extremity; Hand Unit, Department of
Orthopaedic Surgery, University Hospital Vall
d'Hebron, Barcelona, Spain

JOHN A. MARTIN Jr, MD
Medical Director, Commonwealth Sports Medicine; Director of Sports Medicine, St. Joseph Medical Center, Reading, Pennsylvania

DAVID W. MARTINEAU, MD
Former Fellow, Christine M. Kleinert Institute for Hand and Micro Surgery, Louisville, Kentucky; Hand and Upper Extremity Surgeon, The Core Institute, Phoenix, Arizona

ELIZABETH A. MESTER, MS, OTR/L, CHT
Hand Therapy Department, Pennsylvania Hand Center, Bryn Mawr, Pennsylvania

STEVEN L. MORAN, MD
Chief, Division of Plastic Surgery, Mayo Clinic, Rochester, Minnesota

JAMES J. NICHOLSON, MD, MHS
Director, Joint Replacement Center; Assistant Professor, Department of Orthopaedic Surgery, SUNY-Stony Brook Medical Center, Stony Brook, New York

JENNIFER L. REITZ, OTR/L, CHT
Director, Hand Therapy Department, Pennsylvania Hand Center, Bryn Mawr, Pennsylvania

JONATHAN F. ROSENFELD, MD, MBA
Pennsylvania Hand Center; Assistant Professor, Orthopaedic and Hand Surgery, Jefferson Medical College, Philadelphia, Pennsylvania

MARK ROSS, MB, BS, FRACS
Department of Orthopaedic Surgery, Princess Alexandra Hospital; Associate Professor of Orthopaedic Surgery, University of Queensland; Brisbane Hand & Upper Limb Clinic, Brisbane, Queensland, Australia

LUIS R. SCHEKER, MD
Faculty Member, Christine M. Kleinert Institute for Hand and Micro Surgery; Associate Clinical Professor, Division of Plastic and Reconstructive Surgery, School of Medicine, University of Louisville, Louisville, Kentucky

PETER J. STERN, MD
Professor of Orthopaedic Surgery, Department of Orthopaedic Surgery, University of Cincinnati College of Medicine, Cincinnati, Ohio

FRASER TAYLOR, MB, BS, FRACS
Hand and Upper Limb Fellow, Department of Orthopaedic Surgery, Princess Alexandra Hospital; Brisbane Hand & Upper Limb Clinic, Brisbane, Queensland, Australia

MARK A. VITALE, MD, MPH
Hand and Microsurgery Fellow, Department of Orthopaedic Surgery, Rochester, Minnesota

LINDLEY B. WALL, MD
Assistant Professor of Orthopaedic Surgery, Washington University Orthopedics, St Louis, Missouri

MARWAN A. WEHBÉ, MD
Medical Director, Pennsylvania Hand Center, Bryn Mawr, Pennsylvania; Professor Orthopaedic and Hand Surgery, Jefferson Medical College, Philadelphia, Pennsylvania

MARY LEE WHITAKER, RN
Clinical Assistant, Pennsylvania Hand Center, Bryn Mawr, Pennsylvania

Contents

> The history and evolution of both soft tissue and implant arthroplasty about the wrist are discussed, including carpometacarpal, radiocarpal, and distal radioulnar joints. Technical considerations for arthroplasty are reviewed, including factors affecting implant osseointegration, implant articulation/constraint, and management of complications.

> Arthritis at the base of the thumb is common and debilitating. Arthroplasty has evolved over 3 decades to become a highly refined surgical procedure, with excellent results. This article summarizes the history, method, and expected results of basal joint arthroplasty, and the authors describe their method of ligament reconstruction and tendon interposition for thumb basal arthritis.

> The reason there are numerous techniques for thumb carpometacarpal arthroplasty is that none of them are perfect. Sometimes the simplest procedures work best. This article presents a simple alternative, using a readily available suture to stabilize the thumb after resection of the trapezium, with long-term success.

> Trapezium prosthetic arthroplasty has been utilized to treat basal joint arthritis for nearly five decades in an attempt to mitigate some of the potential disadvantages of trapeziectomy while preserving range of motion. Implant arthroplasty seeks to preserve joint biomechanics, avoids metacarpal subsidence, and should provide immediate stability. These benefits may lead to improvements in strength, durability, and a decrease in metacarpophalangeal joint hyperextension which can occur subsequent to metacarpal shortening. First generation implants were primarily silicone trapezial spacers. While the use of these implants has been curtailed by their

association with silicone synovitis, they still remain an option for low demand, rheumatoid patients. More recently developed synthetic spacers such as Artelon interposition arthroplasties have had results inferior to more established procedures including trapeziectomy. A variety of metal total joint prostheses have been developed and some of the more recent designs have shown good short-term outcomes. There are a number of different pyrocarbon implants that have become more recently available which range from trapezial substitution to non-anatomic hemiarthroplasty. Pyrocarbon arthroplasty offers a number theoretical advantages however early results have been mixed and further long term data is required.

Resection arthroplasty is an old, and yet reliable, solution for the isolated osteoarthritis (OA) of some joints of the hand. With complication low rates, this technically undemanding option is ideal for scapho-trapezial-trapezoidal joint OA, as well as for the OA of the carpometacarpal joints of the fingers. This paper reviews its indications, surgical technique, and results.

Proximal row carpectomy (PRC) is a motion-preserving treatment for the degenerated wrist. PRC provides painless wrist range of motion with few complications. PRC treats specifically scapholunate advanced collapse, scaphoid non-union advanced collapse, chronic perilunate dislocations, and Kienbock's disease. The best candidates are older than 35 with an intact capitate head and lunate facet of the distal radius. Proximal row carpectomy provides satisfactory postoperative wrist range of motion and grip strength with few complications, especially when there is no capitolunate arthrosis. Postoperative progressive changes at the radiocapitate articulation have been documented, yet these changes tend to remain asymptomatic.

Although arthrodesis is the treatment preferred by most surgeons for severe wrist arthritis, some degree of functional impairment occurs from the resulting loss of motion, especially when multiple joints in the extremity are affected by arthritis. Total wrist arthroplasty may enhance the performance of daily activities and it is usually preferred by patients over arthrodesis. The newer generation of wrist prostheses has demonstrated improved performance and durability in properly selected patients. This article provides a review of the history, indications, techniques, and outcomes of wrist arthroplasty.

This is a report of the first prosthetic hemiarthroplasty and full arthroplasty, designed and implanted for the distal radioulnar joint in 1988. Two case reports are presented, with follow-up of 24 years. Experience and problems in the design of both a hemiarthroplasty and total prosthetic arthroplasty are described, in the hope that future developments may avoid past failures.

Resection of the ulnar head in cases of debilitating pain owing to arthrosis of the distal radioulnar joint can provide satisfying relief. However, there is mounting evidence that pain with heavier use, instability, and torque-generating weakness in more active individuals may result in less satisfying outcomes. Implant arthroplasty can provide a means to stabilize the radius to the ulna after ulnar head resection, but it requires significant attention to requisite soft tissue stabilization and alignment of the distal radius to the implant to be successful.

This article presents the use of a constrained total distal radioulnar joint replacement with its indications, contraindications, pearls, and pitfalls. The distal radioulnar joint is a complex articulation that carries weight while allowing vector changes without interfering with its function. The total distal radioulnar joint is a solution to those cases with absence of the sigmoid notch, poor soft tissue, or too much ulnar bone resected. The ability of patients to return to regular activities is documented, with a 5-year follow-up.

Hand therapy is essential after arthroplasty around the wrist. This article includes therapy guidelines and goals after surgical reconstruction of the thumb carpometacarpal joint, radiocarpal joint, and distal radioulnar joint. Typical concerns and treatment options are addressed. Tables and figures are included to guide the hand therapist in the process of returning this patient population to pain-free function.

We have searched for a synthetic substitute for the carpal ligaments, which would be widely available and easy to use. Four loops of 2-0 polyester fiber suture (Mersilene) were found to exceed the ultimate tensile strength of the scapholunate interosseous ligament. This construct approximates a normal ligament stress/strain curve and can theoretically facilitate fibrous tissue ingrowth. It is readily available, easy to handle, and inexpensive. Based on these findings, we recommend the use of polyester suture in the reconstruction of carpal and other ligaments.

Carpal ligaments are commonly injured and may lead to pain and disability. These ligaments are very difficult to repair, and the results are unpredictable; as a result, treatment options abound. A novel approach is presented here using a polyester suture, aiming to substitute these ligaments' function, rather than to repair them.

HAND CLINICS

Dedication to Those Who Taught Me

We learn not only from our own successes and failures, but also from the successes and failures of those who preceded us. Anyone we interact with has an influence on our learning process and is an inspiration, including our family, friends, teachers, mentors, students, residents, fellows, hand therapists, nurses; the list goes on…

As I near the latter part of my career, I would like to acknowledge a few of my teachers who had the greatest influence on my career and to whom I will forever be indebted:

Adel Afifi and Ronald Bergman, from my medical school.

Adrian Flatt, Michael Bonfiglio, Ignacio Ponseti, and Reginald Cooper, from my orthopedic residency.

James Hunter and Lawrence Schneider, from my Hand Fellowship.

Ronald Linscheid, James Dobyns, and Harry Buncke, from my postfellowship experience.

I must also include my past and present associates and colleagues, my staff, and my patients with whom each visit is a lesson learned; as well as Robin and Alan, whose dad missed some of their Little League games because of emergency calls!

I like to compare my career to a football game. Past players allowed me to play on their team and helped me carry the ball forward. I hope I have helped move that ball a few yards and passed it to a younger generation, who will carry it further and closer to that goal that seems to be constantly slipping further away.

I would like also to thank the authors in this volume of *Hand Clinics* for their contributions to the subject matter and for taking the time to share their expertise with all of us in this issue, specifically.

Marwan A. Wehbé, MD
Pennsylvania Hand Center
101 S. Bryn Mawr Avenue, Suite 300
Bryn Mawr, PA 19010, USA

E-mail address:
Marwan.Wehbe@pahandcenter.com

http://dx.doi.org/10.1016/j.hcl.2012.09.002
0749-0712/13/$ – see front matter

Foreword

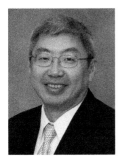

Kevin C. Chung, MD
Consulting Editor

Hand Clinics has been an important educational venue because it provides a rapid dissemination of updated information from the literature in a compact, easy-to-read, review-article format. The topics in *Hand Clinics* were carefully selected to match the new developments in hand surgery as well as to anticipate emerging trends that can shape the future of this specialty. In an effort to consolidate these ideas and to plan future volumes, the management team at *Hand Clinics* will select editors for all of the future clinics series to assure a seamless continuity of updated content. I am excited to be the first Consulting Editor for *Hand Clinics*. I look forward to working with many colleagues in our specialty to provide up-to-date information by leading authors from the United States and around the world. Several upcoming issues of *Hand Clinics* are being organized, including Management of Peripheral Nerve Conditions by Dr Warren Hammert at the University of Rochester, Treatment of Hand Fractures by Dr Jeffrey Lawton, University of Michigan, and Flap Reconstruction of the Upper Extremity by Dr Sandeep Sabastin, National University of Singapore. We would of course be interested in getting new ideas from the hand surgery community to propose topics that are emerging trends in this specialty. These *Hand Clinics* issues strive to provide a quick and updated reference that distills the essence of a topic, making it to everyday practice. I look forward to producing issues that will enhance your library collection.

Kevin C. Chung, MD
Section of Plastic Surgery, Department of Surgery
University of Michigan Medical School
The University of Michigan Health System
2130 Taubman Center
1500 East Medical Center Drive
Ann Arbor, MI 48109, USA

E-mail address:
kecchung@med.umich.edu

http://dx.doi.org/10.1016/j.hcl.2012.09.004
0749-0712/13/$ – see front matter

hand.theclinics.com

Preface

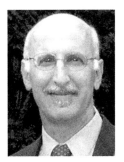

Marwan A. Wehbé, MD
Guest Editor

An arthroplasty is the "repair of a joint." We tend to think of it as joint replacement, although other interventions, such as ligament repair or joint resection, qualify as arthroplasties.

Arthroplasties around the wrist include procedures on the carpometacarpal (CMC) joints, which include both thumb and finger CMC joints, scapho-trapezio-trapezoid (STT), midcarpal (MC), radiocarpal (RC), and distal radioulnar (DRUJ) joints. When we use the term "WRIST," we usually refer to the radiocarpal joint and maybe also the MC joint. For years most publications focused on the wrist; then a period came when the distal radioulnar joint was king. Now all these joints have become somewhat forgotten, so I felt it was time to summarize our knowledge of arthroplasties around the wrist. Past and present solutions have solved many problems, as our knowledge expanded, but do we know it all yet?

This publication is the ideal medium to summarize knowledge to date and to report studies on the edge of scientific progress. Peer review is limited here and provides the reader with topic updates and the raw materials that allow one to decide on the merits of a study. Aside from providing updates on a topic, this should challenge and stimulate the reader toward further research and development.

Assessment and reporting of results still lag behind advances in our knowledge. Grip strength is often reported in kilograms, while scientific publications thrive to use the metric system (SI). In the metric system, however, kilogram is a unit of mass, not force. The equivalent SI unit of force is the newton (N). One newton is the amount of force required to give a 1 kg mass an acceleration of 1 m/s/s. In the English system, the pound (lbs) happens to be a unit of mass as well as of force. Therefore grip should be reported in newtons or pounds, not in kilograms!

Most studies report grip strength as a percentage of the contralateral hand. Considering that the dominant hand is 10% stronger in a right-handed person and equal in the 2 hands of a left-handed person, using the percentage of the uninjured side conveys no useful information.[1] Outcome reports should use a percentage of predicted grip strength rather than a comparison to the contralateral side.

Range of motion reporting contains an equally flawed premise. There is no agreement on how to measure range of motion for any joint. Measurements by estimation, by use of a caliper, or by radiographs will result in a great discrepancy on a particular joint, based on the examiner's technique, swelling, or deformity around the joint being measured. The thumb CMC joint is the most difficult to measure because of its capacity to move in multiple axes in space. All we can hope for is consistency within each study, which is rarely achieved, considering that multiple examiners

Hand Clin 29 (2013) xiii–xiv
http://dx.doi.org/10.1016/j.hcl.2012.09.003

hand.theclinics.com

are recording their findings, obtained by different methods.

Some journals reject reports that do not use statistical tools extensively. This is unfortunate, because novel ideas and methods need to be shared with a wide audience to stimulate progress. Not all scientific information is subject to statistics. This reminds me of publications that collect surveys, based on subject recollections, and then apply extensive statistics to the results. These "statistically significant" results are based on data collected by guesswork and estimation! Garbage in, garbage out.

Marwan A. Wehbé, MD
Pennsylvania Hand Center
101 S. Bryn Mawr Avenue, Suite 300
Bryn Mawr, PA 19010, USA

E-mail address:
Marwan.Wehbe@pahandcenter.com

REFERENCE

1. Crosby CA, Wehbé MA. Hand strength normative values. J Hand Surg 1994;19A:665–70.

History and Design Considerations for Arthroplasty Around the Wrist

Jonathan F. Rosenfeld, MD, MBA[a],*,
James J. Nicholson, MD, MHS[b]

KEYWORDS

- Total wrist arthroplasty • History • Carpometacarpal arthroplasty • Implant • Osseointegration
- Biomaterials

KEY POINTS

- The history and evolution of both soft tissue and implant arthroplasty about the wrist are discussed, including carpometacarpal radiocarpal, and distal radioulnar joints.
- Technical considerations for arthroplasty are reviewed, including factors affecting implant osseointegration, implant articulation/constraint, and management of complications.
- The wrist contains many joints, each of which can degenerate and become painful, leading to overall loss of function of the upper extremity.

INTRODUCTION

Arthroplasty is defined as surgical reconstruction of a diseased joint. The wrist contains many joints, each of which can degenerate and become painful, leading to overall loss of function of the upper extremity. Treatment of painful or problematic joints about the wrist has been a part of medicine for centuries. As anatomic knowledge expanded, the source of disability became clearer and treatments were developed to address specific areas. Each anatomic area has it own history; treatment methodology is shared between anatomic knowledge of joint interrelationships and advances in technology.

HISTORY OF COMMON ARTHROPLASTIES AROUND THE WRIST
Thumb Carpometacarpal Joint

Arthrosis at the thumb carpometacarpal joint is common and disabling. The history of treatment of this condition is interesting in that it is not linear. Many of the described and tested techniques are still in use or regaining favor. Although many procedures have been used to treat this common disease, most have their root in excision of all or part of the trapezium bone. Often the difference between procedures is the reconstruction, if any, that occurs after the bone is removed. However, unlike some other joints, there also exist procedures designed to treat the joint before the point of full painful degeneration. Rather than salvage, these reconstructive procedures are aimed at preventing or at least delaying the onset of painful degeneration of the joint and are a step past simple joint debridement, open or arthroscopic.

The pathology of thumb carpometacarpal degeneration is theorized to relate to failure of the ligamentous stabilizers of the joint, especially the anterior oblique (volar beak) ligament. For this reason, reconstructions of these ligaments, often involving tendon harvest, have been used to stall progression of degeneration and avoid trapezium

Funding sources: Dr Rosenfeld: None. Dr Nicholson: Implant royalties, Kinamed Inc. Conflicts of interest: Dr Rosenfeld: None. Dr Nicholson: None.
[a] Orthopedic and Hand Surgery, Jefferson Medical College, Philadelphia, PA, USA; [b] Joint Replacement Center, Department of Orthopedic Surgery, SUNY-Stony Brook Medical Center, HSC T18, R80, Stony Brook, NY 11790, USA
* Corresponding author.
E-mail address: jonathan.rosenfeld@pahandcenter.com

hand.theclinics.com

excision.[1-3] Results for early-stage degeneration have been favorable. To treat early degeneration at the proximal end of the trapezium at the same setting, a double stabilization procedure is required.[4]

Another technique that preserves the trapezium is osteotomy of the thumb metacarpal, changing the alignment of the joint.[5-7] This procedure has a long history, with variable frequency of use over the decades. Metacarpal extension is gained through performing a closing wedge osteotomy at the dorsal base of the thumb metacarpal. This procedure alters the contact forces to avoid the typical wear at the volar ulnar aspect of the thumb metacarpal base. Results have been favorable in early stages of disease, but technique acceptance has been variable. This procedure has the advantage of maintaining all other future treatment options. However, it does not address pain emanating from degeneration at the scaphotrapezial-trapezoid (STT) joint.

As with many other joints, arthrodesis is a treatment option for degeneration of the thumb carpometacarpal joint; any existing degeneration of the STT joint is not treated with CMC arthrodesis. With fusion all carpometacarpal joint motion is lost, unlike the other options available for thumb carpometacarpal degeneration. This loss of motion is theoretically traded for increased stability and ability to perform high-demand tasks. Functional deficit, related to lost motion at the thumb carpometacarpal joint, has not been definitively proven. For many years, arthrodesis was the option taught and selected for the manual laborer. Success is also seen in the older patient. Nonunion, however, is a risk not seen with other treatment techniques. Regardless of the technique used to obtain fusion, results of multiple studies have not provided conclusive outcomes.[8-10]

Remaining options for arthroplasty of the thumb carpometacarpal joint involve removing all or part of the trapezium, either open or arthroscopically. Gervis[11] described in 1948 the excision of the trapezium for carpometacarpal degeneration. In his follow-up paper, he notes that the procedure had been performed "hundreds" of times and that the results with 30 years' experience were "entirely satisfactory."[12] In fact, he underwent the procedure himself when the pain "made operating tiring and hobbies distasteful." He notes the still-present lengthy recovery: "winding clocks was irksome and it was a year before a clock with a strong spring could be wound." Around the same time, Murley[13] also noted good results with simple trapezium excision.

Excision of the entire trapezium is often followed by a procedure to fill the bone's void. This process theoretically decreases subsidence/shortening of

the ray and could provide increased grip strength. Swanson[14] developed a silicone implant to replace the trapezium in the 1960s. Good initial relief was seen, but rates of long-term complication were high, including synovitis, subluxation, and bony erosion.[15] The technique as described is rarely performed. However, many other implants exist to fill the void when a trapezium has been fully or partially excised.

The Artelon spacer, shaped like a letter T and made of theoretically degradable polyurethane-urea, promised to create an ingrowth of fibrocartilage to cover the excised distal surface of the trapezium.[16] Although stronger pinch strengths have occasionally been noted in the short term, long-term evidence did not show the Artelon to be superior to trapezium excision with or without a ligament stabilization procedure.[17] Additionally, several patients have required revision to more traditional arthroplasty to obtain functional improvement and pain relief.

Multiple total and hemi joint arthroplasty systems have been marketed. Many of these were removed from production because of loosening, subluxation, or need for revision. When comparing any technique with simple bone excision, cost is also a factor, especially when the outcome cannot be proven to be superior. Additionally, both pyrocarbon and ball-and-socket metal-and-plastic designs are still available for use today. In both of these designs, a portion of the trapezium is excised and the implant's stem is inserted into the metacarpal. The long-term results of these implants are not yet known.[18-21]

A tendon, often palmaris longus and later flexor carpi radialis, has been used to fill the void left by the partially or completely resected trapezium.[22] A combination of ligament reconstruction and tendon interposition (LRTI) was described by Burton and Pellegrini.[23] Initially, they compared this technique with silicone implants in their 2-part article. Multiple variations on the LRTI theme were introduced since, and many are still in use, including using first dorsal compartment tendons or the palmaris longus.[24] Recently, nonautologous material has been used for ligament reconstruction after trapezium excision. Some examples are Mersilene tape and suture anchors or buttons.

Today the LRTI is considered by some to be the gold-standard procedure for thumb carpometacarpal arthritis, but that standard is being challenged. Recent studies have questioned the need for reconstructing the ligament or pinning the joint space after excising the trapezium openly[25,26] or arthroscopically.[27] This debate demonstrates the nonlinear progression of treatment for this condition. Davis and colleagues[28] compared trapezium excision with no reconstruction, tendon interposition (palmaris longus), and ligament reconstruction with the flexor carpi radialis. At 1 year, good results were seen with all methods, with no statistically significant difference. Another study[29] noted no need for prolonged (4 weeks) postoperative immobilization after simple trapezium excision when comparing results in the short term.

Thumb carpometacarpal degenerative disease is common and disabling. A large arsenal of treatment options has both grown and shrunk over the course of history. Clearly, the history and best option for carpometacarpal arthroplasty has yet to be fully elucidated.

The Wrist (Radiocarpal Joint)

Painful degeneration of the wrist from infection, trauma, or systemic conditions will limit the function of the upper extremity. Arthroplasty of the radiocarpal joint is not a recent event, although the progression of research is more rapid and options are more varied today than ever before. Initial treatment for severe infection was amputation which, although lifesaving, was clearly a functional deficit. As medical treatment evolved centuries ago, resection of the damaged joint led to a salvaged hand with limited function. This function would increase as the wrist stiffened, although pain was still a factor.

Formal arthrodesis of the wrist joint for infection, painful degeneration, or malalignment predates the modern medical era of asepsis and anesthesia, and is still a viable option in the current arsenal. Many different techniques have been discussed to achieve fusion.[30–34] Placing the hand in a functional position and making it stable and without pain are critical to the functional success of this procedure regardless of the technique. Total wrist fusion, generally accepted as fusion between the radius, lunate, capitate, and often the third metacarpal, provides these requisites. Modifications may be needed depending on the specific abnormality or desire for increased fusion mass.

In addition to total fusion of the wrist, limited or partial wrist fusions have also been popular.[35] In theory, these procedures will yield the requisite stability and absence of pain, and can maintain some functional arc of motion.

STT fusion[36,37] has been described in many articles as a treatment for degeneration and carpal collapse. Although the arthrodesis rates and results are not always consistent among reports, biomechanical and clinical studies of this partial fusion have aided the development of additional fusion procedures to relieve pain and increase function. Scaphocapitate fusion was described in 1946[38] for scaphoid nonunion. Additional cases were described in 1952.[39] In 1991, this procedure was reviewed at an average of 2 years postoperatively in 17 patients.[40] There were two nonunions and 7 patients had mild to moderate pain with heavy use.

More central in the wrist, the fusion of the lunate to the capitate without involving the radius produces a carpus similar to a total fusion but preserves motion at the radiocarpal joint.[41,42] Initially this "4-corner" fusion involved the lunate, capitate, hamate, and triquetrum. More recently, fusion of just the lunate to the capitate, with or without excision of the triquetrum, has been performed.[43] The scaphoid is excised in each method. Separately, when the disease is limited to the radiocarpal joint, without severe midcarpal disease or malalignment, fusion of the radius to the lunate or the scaphoid and lunate is an option.[42,44]

Arthrodesis for wrist degeneration is no longer the panacea it was once believed to be. It remains, however, viable as either an initial treatment option or salvage for failed total wrist arthroplasty.

A salvage option that remains popular today and does not require healing of a fusion is the proximal row carpectomy. Excision of the scaphoid, lunate, and triquetrum creates a joint between the capitate head and the lunate facet of the distal radius. In most cases of wrist degeneration from scaphoid nonunion or scapholunate ligament abnormality, this lunate facet is spared degeneration. In theory, but not always in reality, without existing degeneration of the capitate head, the new articulation should remain free of degeneration and provide a functional wrist with decreased pain. The results of this longstanding procedure have been variable but generally positive.[45–47]

Compared with many other joints, artificial wrist joints came into use at a much later stage, mostly because fusion was the accepted treatment for end-stage painful wrists. Because the pain was relieved with the fusion, less incentive existed to investigate replacement of the joint. Despite the recent progression to what is considered typical total wrist arthroplasty, arthroplasties about the wrist have a long history. Aside from fusion (both partial and complete), resection arthroplasty was likely the first form of wrist arthroplasty to relieve pain and maintain motion. Resection arthroplasty of joints is known to have occurred many years ago, even before the advent of anesthesia. Attempts to excise joints while maintaining distal motion were recorded as early as 1536.[48,49] These reports include a resection arthroplasty for infection of the elbow joint by Ambroise Paré. Specific to the wrist, the reported first account of wrist joint resection was in 1762 by Johann Ulrich Beyer.[48,49] The procedure was well documented; it was performed for trauma and subsequent infection. The reported result was a natural-looking hand with limited function. Although the goal of this procedure was not specifically an arthrodesis, a wrist with little motion was a significant improvement over amputation.

Further reports on wrist joint resection, followed by immobilization resulting in ankylosis or pseudoankylosis were reported at the end of the 18th century. Moreau and his son reported the data to the French Academy of surgeons and published a book about this technique[48]; these surgeons, however, did not receive credit for their contributions to wrist arthroplasty and its importance was not realized at that time.[49] John Rhea Barton from the University of Pennsylvania is credited as having performed the first wrist arthroplasty in 1826.[48] It is reported that he specifically emphasized early mobilization in an effort to avoid ankylosis. As anesthesia became more prevalent, multiple surgeons performed additional resection arthroplasties. These were often performed for tuberculosis or trauma. Early mobilization became a goal and was performed by the likes of Syme, White, and Park.[48] Toward that end, recommendations were made to perform the dissection subperiosteally, which led to recommendations for interposition arthroplasty. Multiple versions of interposition arthroplasty for the wrist and multiple other joints have been used over the years. Interposition arthroplasty remains an option for treatment of joint degeneration. In the late 1800s many materials were tested for interposition, including adipose tissue, skin, glass, pig bladder, rubber, gold foil, and fascia.[49] With the current medical knowledge and status of arthroplasty, interposition arthroplasty is used much less frequently but can still be a useful alternative in a difficult situation.

Noting the failure of interposition of the above-noted materials, and out of a desire to maintain motion and function, the concept of total wrist replacement was born. Thermistocles Gluck (1853–1942) is credited as having designed the first true total wrist arthroplasty.[49,50] He experimented with a variety of materials, including bone cement. He performed a total knee arthroplasty with ivory in 1890 and an ivory total wrist arthroplasty in the same year. This device consisted of 2 "forks" that inserted into the proximal and distal part of the joint with an ivory component in the center. Unfortunately, Gluck was shunned by other members of the Berlin medical community and was unable to present his research and

results. In 1891, he ended up being forced to admit failure of the arthroplasty because of the development of a chronic discharging sinus from tuberculosis, despite the patient's having functional range of motion at 1-year follow-up. Eventually, he was able to report on long-term results of his implants in 1921.[49,50]

Over the ensuing half-century, research focused on implant materials such as glass and Vitallium.[48,49] This research was conducted mainly on hip and knee arthroplasties. The volume of research on hip and knee arthroplasty continues to outpace that of wrist arthroplasty, and this parallels the volume of implant arthroplasties being performed. Experimentation on wrist arthroplasty continued, including research on hinged-type designs and interpositional spacing. John Niebauer[51] and Alfred Swanson[52–54] researched interpositional spacers made of silicone. This evaluation initially focused on interphalangeal joints, but implants were also developed for the radiocarpal joint in 1967. The goal of the interpositional spacer was to provide stability while maintaining range of motion to allow the formation of a fibrous tissue sleeve; this capsule would then provide functional motion and stability. Unfortunately, although initial results revealed good pain relief and acceptable motion, the implants tended to break or subside. When combined with silicone synovitis, the implants did not provide a long-term viable solution.[55–58]

In 1969, Gschwend and Scheier implanted the Gschwend-Scheier-Bähler wrist. In 1972, Hans Christoph Meuli[59] introduced a prosthesis he designed. He noted that, because the center of movement of the wrist joint is closely consistent with the head of the capitate, the ball-and-socket-type joint should reproduce all of the required motions of the wrist. His design was not unlike Gluck's, with fork-like pegs heading in both proximal and distal directions. Each component had 2 pegs. A polyester ball sat between the components, held in place by the shape of the metal components and giving 3° of freedom. These pegs were bendable and were implanted into the metacarpals and the radius with methyl methacrylate. Meuli noted improved mechanical alignment when implanting into the second and third metacarpals rather than the third and fourth. In addition to the radial carpus, the distal ulna and radial styloid were resected in this technique. Complications included subsidence, migration, loss of fixation, and ulnar deviation of the hand.

Around the same time, in 1974, Voltz[60,61] designed an implant with a single proximal stem made of cobalt-chrome and included a polyethylene articular surface. Distally, the implant remained double-stemmed. Unlike complete ball-and-socket motion, this was restricted to mainly 2° of freedom (flexion-extension and radial-ulnar deviation) by the design of the implant. This implant and others, such as the Guepar,[62] also suffered similar failures of loosening and malalignment of the hand.[63] Wear of the components themselves has been less of an issue for the wrist than for the lower extremities.

In an effort to correct the noted issues, new prostheses were created as variations on the above designs. Staff at the Mayo Clinic designed the biaxial total wrist.[64] Five-year follow-up analysis of 46 implants for rheumatoid arthritis revealed that 62% of patients felt much better and 75% reported no pain; 11 failures (17%) were reported, 8 of which were distal component loosening. Many patients required revision procedures over the period that this implant was on the market. Some were revised to fusion and others to arthroplasty again.[65] Although initial data were somewhat promising and modifications to the implant were made,[66] this implant eventually was removed from the market because of continued issues with distal stem loosening and radial subsidence.

In the past 10 to 15 years, implant design has focused on limited bony resection, especially of the distal radius, to help offset the subsidence and deviation. Resection of the ulna is no longer part of the wrist arthroplasty implant technique. Additional modifications and designs continued to surface to deal with issues of stability, strength of fixation, range of motion, limitations on migration, and alignment.

Most recent total wrist designs are press-fit/bone-ingrowth materials rather than cemented. In all cases, the head of the capitate remains the center of rotation. Menon[67] designed the Universal wrist implant, a nonconstrained titanium implant with an ingrowth stem and a 20° inclination of the radial component. The carpal component is held with 3 screws and a polyethylene insert is attached to it. This design has been revised, with a deeper radial componentry and larger screws for the distal component.[68] The resection of the radius required for implantation has also been reduced. In addition to this Universal II implant, the RE-MOTION total wrist arthroplasty (SBi [Small Bone Innovations, Inc., 505 Park Avenue, 14th Floor, New York]) is designed to limit radial resection while preserving centralization of the wrist.[69] This implant also preserves ligamentous structures, which add stability and preserve the distal radioulnar joint (DRUJ).

Currently, total wrist implants are available from SBi, Integra (Kineticos Medical, Inc.), Biomet, and others. Additionally, current designs allow for hemiarthroplasty of the wrist at the radiocarpal joint and DRUJ. Results from these recent-generation implants are more promising. Surgical indications have widened as the results have improved.

DRUJ

Arthroplasty and reconstruction of the DRUJ is performed for a variety of indications, including degeneration, instability, and ulnar impingement. Each indication has its own procedural history.

Degeneration of the DRUJ is less common than radiocarpal or thumb carpometacarpal degeneration and may be caused by posttraumatic, osteoarthritic, or rheumatoid disease. The initial treatment for DRUJ degeneration was excision of the head of the ulna. Although described by Darrach in 1912[70] and 1936 and often attributed to him, it was actually described and performed more than 3 decades earlier.[71] Many articles and technique recommendations have followed, describing subperiosteal dissection and length of ulna to be excised. Distal ulna resection, although still used today in certain situations, leaves many issues untreated, including DRUJ instability, ulnar shift of the carpus, and ulnar stump impingement onto the radius. In an effort to address these issues, Bowers[72] designed the hemiresection-interposition procedure. Instead of removing the entire ulnar head, only the articular portion is removed with a saw or osteotome. Various interposition techniques have also been described. One must be cautious of instability of the DRUJ and impingement between the remaining ulna (styloid) and the carpus. A variation on this theme is the burred and rounded matched resection by Watson and colleagues.[73] This procedure also preserves the styloid and DRUJ while removing the articular surface of the ulna head.

In 1936, Sauvé and Kapandji[74] presented another option for DRUJ degeneration. Rather then excise the ulnar head, the head was fused at the DRUJ and an osteotomy was made proximally through the neck. This osteotomy would progress to pseudoarthrosis, allowing forearm rotation without motion at the DRUJ while providing ulnar carpal support.[75] Results have generally been satisfactory despite reports of instability of the ulnar stump.

Ulnocarpal impingement can be treated by a variety of procedures about the DRUJ. Most involve shortening the ulna in some fashion. Formal diaphyseal ulnar shortening, first described by Milch[76] in 1942, can decrease the impingement and theoretically tighten the ulnocarpal ligaments. As with all osteotomies, nonunion/malunion is an associated risk. Shortening can also be of benefit if the radius has been shortened (eg, posttraumatic), leaving the DRUJ incongruent; through shortening the ulna to match the radius, the ulnar head is reseated in the sigmoid notch of the radius. Many variations on the osteotomy itself have been described and several specific plating and osteotomy systems for this procedure are now available, although the plate design may not be critical to the success of the operation.[77]

In an effort to decrease ulnocarpal impaction without the increased complication of a diaphyseal osteotomy, Feldon and colleagues[78] described a distal ulna wafer resection. In this procedure, 2 to 4 mm of distal ulnar head is resected while preserving adjacent soft tissues. Currently, this is can be performed arthroscopically, but it obviously does not address any DRUJ problems.

In addition to arthritis of the DRUJ and ulnocarpal impingement, instability of the DRUJ (both acute and chronic) leads to pain and impaired function. The stabilizing structures of the DRUJ are complex and include the osseous stability of the sigmoid notch, triangular fibrocartilage complex (TFC), extensor carpi ulnaris subsheath, and DRUJ ligaments. If the issue is the competency of the sigmoid notch, an osteoplasty can be performed. The TFC may be repairable. Procedures to address stability of the intact or excised ulnar head have included soft tissue reconstructions, tendon stabilization procedures, and implants. In 2002, Adams and Berger[79] published a technique to reconstruct the anatomic origin and insert the dorsal and volar radioulnar ligaments using a palmaris longus or plantaris tendon weaved through drill holes in the radius and ulna.

As with other joints about the wrist, Swanson[80] developed a silicone implant for the DRUJ. Silicone synovitis, implant failure, and poor long-term results lead to failure of this design.[81] True arthroplasty or joint replacement of the distal radial ulnar joint can remove the unpredictability of soft tissue reconstruction while providing a painless site of load transfer and removing radioulnar impingement. Wehbé[82] described this technique in 1991, and implants are still evolving but have shown good promise. Options for joint replacement include partial or complete ulnar head replacement or total DRUJ replacement, either constrained or unconstrained.

An ulnar head implant is useful for early and late joint reconstructions. Variations exist in the modularity and materials, but generally the results have been promising for hemiarthroplasty with a stem in the ulna. Materials include cobalt-chrome and pyrocarbon. These press-fit designs generally have adjustable-size heads, stems, and necks to accommodate anatomy and revision procedures. Stability of the DRUJ can be gained via soft tissue reconstruction around or sometimes into the implant (holes provided). A sigmoid notch replacement is also currently on the market that, when combined with the ulnar head prosthesis, creates an unconstrained total DRUJ replacement. Definitive data on the benefit of hemiarthroplasty versus total arthroplasty for the DRUJ are not yet available. Also available is the semiconstrained ball-and-socket total DRUJ replacement designed by Shecker.[83] Long-term results have yet to be described, but intermediate results have been promising.

The history of arthroplasty about the wrist is clearly still being written. Significant advances have been made in the past few decades. As of now, definitive data on the best implant, timing, rehabilitation, restrictions, and indications are limited but growing.

THEORETICAL CONSIDERATIONS

When discussing the implant choices around the wrist, each of the potential joint reconstructions (carpometacarpal, radiocarpal, and DRUJ) must be examined separately because of their unique kinematics and the individual functions they serve. This section does not focus on a single joint but serves as a general review of the concepts necessary for successful modern joint replacement and reviews potential limitations of the wrist as a site for joint replacement.

Implant Fixation

Except for the carpometacarpal joint, for which soft tissue–integrating or space-filling inert materials may be chosen, the success of other joint replacements begins with implant fixation. Long-term fixation of implants can be achieved in 2 ways: mechanical fixation through cementing or osseointegration of the implant–bone interface.

Early designs used cement to achieve immediate fixation of implants. Hip arthroplasty fixation with cement is successful because minimal distraction forces are present at the interface. The cement can act on a smooth finished stem like a grouting to achieve fixation. The wrist has torsional and distraction forces, and therefore smooth stems are likely to fail with common distraction through activities of daily living. However if the stem surface is roughened, this may lead to cracking of the interface and generation of cement debris, ultimately leading to loosening of the implant construct.[84] At the bone–cement interface, cement fixation requires adequate cancellous bone to achieve a microlock of the cement.[85] Distal fixation into the carpus and metacarpals in early-generation wrist arthroplasties failed because of a combination of poor bone quality and distraction and torsional forces imparted on the bone–cement interface.[63] Similar failures of cemented total knees and revision hip arthroplasty have been seen when the quality of the cancellous bone is too poor for the cement to achieve interdigitation.[86,87] Because of these modes of failure, cement fixation is unlikely to be the choice for modern implant arthroplasty designs around the wrist.

Osseointegration is the direct structural and functional connection between ordered living bone and the surface of a load-carrying implant. Successful integration of metal implants and bone depends on a proper understanding of material science, host bone biology, and joint kinematics.

Implant-related factors

Most implant designs use cobalt-chrome, titanium, or (less often) pyrocarbon implanted into the cancellous bone to achieve osseointegration. Cobalt-based alloys are highly resistant to corrosion because of their spontaneous formation of a passive oxide layer.[88] They have very high resistance to fatigue and excellent wear resistance against polyethylene.[89] Titanium alloys similarly form a protective oxide layer against corrosion.[88] Although their resistance to fatigue is lower than the cobalt alloys, the relatively low loads that wrist implants endure will unlikely challenge their ultimate strength.[88] Another limitation of titanium alloys is their poor wear characteristics compared with polyethylene.[90] The advantages of titanium over chromium include enhanced biocompatibility to host bone, more moderate elastic modulus, and improved integration to bone.[91]

Pyrocarbon is a less frequently chosen material for implants requiring osseointegration. Because of its biologic compatibility against host bone and its modulus of elasticity closer to that of bone, it is less likely to lead to stress shielding and bone resorption from modulus mismatch.[92] Like cobalt-chrome, pyrocarbon implants act more favorably against host cartilage than titanium alloys, and therefore may do well in hemiarthroplasty designs that rest against host cartilage.[93] However, the clinical success of this material may be challenged by its inferior osseointegrative properties, especially in joints that see high loads or distraction forces.[93]

Material surface factors

Implants can be divided into roughened surface-coated implants (eg, titanium hydroxyapatite or plasma-sprayed) or implants with roughened surfaces without a coating (eg, sand-blasted, acid-etched, or anodically roughened). Roughened surfaces increase the contact area for direct osteoblast attachment and enhance the subsequent bone proliferation and differentiation.[94,95] Most of these surfaces achieve ongrowth and not true ingrowth. Three-dimensional porous metals made of titanium and tantalum are currently available, which can be either attached to the current implants or possibly manufactured in the proper shapes to improve deeper penetration of the osseointegration. These materials would have to be developed with the appropriate 100- to 500-μm pore size, which has been shown to be the optimal range for osseointegration.[96,97]

Initial mechanical stability

During the first few weeks, initial implant stability must be achieved through a solid mechanical wedging or peg/screw fixation of the implant against bone. Minimal micromotion (<50–100 μm) and gaps (<50 μm) must be present at the implant–bone interface for osseointegration to occur.[98] The initial mechanical fixation must remain stable during this biologic integration stage; if excessive micromotion or gaps are present, then the initial mechanical fixation will fail and unstable fibrous ingrowth of the implant and ultimate failure will occur. Initial mechanical stability must be both axially and torsionally stable. This stability is potentially enhanced through wedging anatomically shaped implants into the corticocancellous bone envelope or placing ingrowth pegs or screws, or using a combination of these techniques. Other enhancements in mechanical stability will be achieved through continued refinement of surgical instrumentation that will make bone preparation more facile and reliable. Further development of different sizes and more anatomic shaping of the implants will also enhance the initial stability of the implant, allowing biologic osseointegration to occur.

Host bone factors

One of the limiting factors to success in implant arthroplasty around the wrist is the poor quality of the host bone. Many patients experience disuse osteopenia, inflammatory erosions, senile osteoporosis, or a combination of these issues. Good results have been seen in achieving bone integration of ingrowth in the distal radius component of the radiocarpal replacements.[99] This success is because larger anatomically designed implants can be properly wedged into even poor-quality bone. These results are in contrast to many of the other fixation locations around the wrist, such as the first metacarpal (in a carpometacarpal arthroplasty) and distal carpus (total wrist arthroplasty).[100] The success in these areas has been challenged because of the short length of stems or pegs in pathologic bone. If the quality of the bone is not optimal for osseointegration, attention should be given not to further decrease the vascularity of the bone during the procedure. Continued refinement of the instrumentation will enable the procedure to be performed with less soft tissue stripping.

Potential adjuvants

With the wrist being a challenging area in which to achieve stable osseointegration, some potential measures could increase the chance of success. A cancellous bone graft from the prepared bone may be used to fill gaps or erosions. Osteoinductive hydroxyapatite may also be used to coat implants to enhance the apposition of bone.[101,102] Because of the superficial nature of the arthroplasties around the wrist, biophysical stimulation may be possible to enhance the osseointegration of implants.[103] Further research using either pulsed electromagnetic fields or low-intensity pulsed ultrasound must be performed.

Implant Articulation

For each of the joints around the wrist, data support both hemiarthroplasty and total arthroplasty. A hemiarthroplasty is fixed to bone on one side and articulates with host cartilage. Host cartilage has been shown to prefer articulation against pyrocarbon and cobalt-chrome alloys compared with titanium alloys; however, the success of the pyrocarbon implants may be limited to low-load joints (carpometacarpal) because of their poor ingrowth characteristics compared with cobalt alloys.[90–92] Although the hemiarthroplasty may improve clinical outcomes early, it is at risk of developing wear at the articulating cartilage and subsequent subsidence into the host bone. In contrast, a total arthroplasty will have implants fixed on either side of the joint with an articulating surface. Their success will be limited by the difficult initial stability and subsequent osseointegration into the carpus.[104]

Whether the carpometacarpal or the radiocarpal joint is being addressed, the area of challenging fixation is the carpal component, which is why renewed interest has been seen in returning to a less complicated hemiarthroplasty. If future implant designs can improve the success of carpal implant integration, long-term success may then favor the total joint arthroplasty over the hemiarthroplasty. Recent issues with metal-on-metal hip articulation generating metal inflammatory debris or metal hypersensitivity has returned metal-on-plastic to the bearing of choice.[105,106] In addition, wear of articulating plastic has not been a significant issue in arthroplasties around the wrist. The hip literature has also shown that cobalt alloy articulation with plastic is superior to titanium alloy on plastic. Therefore, the surface of future total implants will likely be cobalt alloy on polyethylene.

Implant Constraint/Balance

Increasing constraint of any implant design is well understood to lead to increased stress at the implant-bone interface, thereby leading to earlier failures from aseptic loosening or fracture. An obvious example of this would be the older total wrist designs, which were fully constrained.[107] Unconstrained or partially constrained implants therefore constitute most currently available designs. These implants rely on proper soft tissue balancing to achieve proper kinematics of the joint.[108] Proper implant kinematics depend on functional tendons, preserved joint capsule, and articulation centers as close to the native position as possible.

Patient Selection

Patients for whom soft tissue reconstructions of the carpometacarpal or DRUJ failed may be appropriate for implant arthroplasty if their remaining bone stock is appropriate.[109] Until improved long-term outcomes of radiocarpal arthroplasty are confirmed, this surgery should be reserved for older patients with low functional demands but adequate bone stock, especially those with bilateral radiocarpal arthritis. Malnutrition and/or a history of infection, poor vascularity, or inadequate bone stock are absolute contraindications to wrist arthroplasty.[110]

Patients who use nicotine products should be told to stop during the perioperative period. Some medications may also adversely affect wound healing and osseointegration.[111] The surgeon must examine the patient's medication list for disease-modifying antirheumatic drugs, nonsteroidal anti-inflammatory drugs, and corticosteroids. Preoperative consultation with the patient's primary care provider or rheumatologist may be needed to limit or eliminate these medications during the perioperative period to improve success.

Duration of Immobilization

Current postoperative motion protocols are variable and have limited scientific support. Early splinting has many benefits. It allows improved initial stability of the implants, which will enhance osseointegration of the implant. It will protect microfractures (that occurred during implant seating/preparation) from propagating and allows soft tissue healing, which may decrease the incidence of infection. It may also decrease the risk of dislocation through allowing healing of the soft tissue envelope that was violated during surgery. Further research is needed to understand when these benefits will be outweighed by the negative outcomes of ultimate postoperative range of motion, recovery time, and patient satisfaction.

Periprosthetic Infection

Proper patient selection and preparation are the initial steps in avoiding a postoperative infection.[112] Patients with prior infections of that wrist, poor skin envelope, poor vascularity of the hand, or malnutrition must be avoided. Healthy wound healing will be improved with appropriate skin preparation, timely antibiotic prophylaxis, minimal soft tissue trauma during surgery, and immobilization of the soft tissues for a period after surgery. The combination of older age with rheumatoid arthritis and medications, and the thin soft tissue envelope covering the implants, is unfortunately associated with a significant incidence of infection. Continued swelling, warmth, and pain may serve as clinical signs to evaluate for a potentially deep infection.

In patients with noninflammatory arthritis, an erythrocyte sedimentation rate or C-reactive protein may be a good initial screening test. Aspiration of the joint fluid may be sent for culture. For acute infections (within 4 weeks of surgery), an open irrigation and debridement of the joint can be attempted. Carpometacarpal spacer implants should be removed or replaced. Implants fixed to bone will remain with exchange of any modular parts. The patient will then be placed on appropriate antibiotics for 4 to 6 weeks. Chronic (>4 weeks) infections have 2 options: (1) open irrigation of implants and soft tissue with organism-specific antibiotic suppression attempted for life, or (2) removal of implants and any foreign bodies with a goal of full eradication of the infection. Until further studies are performed, definitive treatment of a chronic deep infection will need to follow the history of other joint replacement sites.[113] After implants are removed, a high-dose antibiotic spacer can be left to stabilize the soft tissues and introduce a high dose of antibiotics into the area. The patient will be treated with 4 to 6 weeks of antibiotics. Once antibiotics are discontinued, the inflammatory markers should remain stable for 3 to 4 weeks. A salvage procedure of choice will then be performed.

Periprosthetic Fracture Management

Like other joint replacements, the treatment of fractures will depend on where the fracture is and whether the implant is stable (fixed through osseointegration or cement into bone). For implants with stable fixation, the surgeon must evaluate if the fracture is likely to heal with traditional immobilization. If this is not possible or it fails, then open surgical procedures will need to be performed. Proximal fractures around radius and ulna components are fixed with traditional open plating techniques. More complex challenges will exist in the hand portion of the implant. Extensive carpal–metacarpal fusions may enhance the stability of these difficult distal fractures. Fractures occurring around loose implant fixation must be treated with salvage options.

Salvage Options

Failed arthroplasties can be salvaged with conventional fusion, resection, and/or interpositional techniques. Conversion to a fusion may be difficult.[114] The poor bone stock available will make this a challenging endeavor for any surgeon. Proper length of the wrist must be maintained to allow adequate motion and strength. Previous case reports have documented some success with the use of structural allografts (eg, femoral head) with complex fixation techniques.[115] However, allografts have minimal integration to the host bone and have a high risk of absorption, infection, and delayed fracture. Vascular bone autografts may also be a option.[116] Strong 3-dimensional porous metals may help salvage these difficult cases in the future.[117] These metals can be designed or intraoperatively shaped to fit a defined defect. Further development and research of this area is needed.

Revision radiocarpal arthroplasty can also be attempted. Although it may seem like an attractive choice to use longer cemented implants in a revision, these are likely to fail. Revision of the loose arthroplasty will need to be performed with more complex osseointegrative components. Loose radius implants can be handled with a more extensively coated and longer radial revision implant design.[118] The more likely and challenging case will be the revision of the loose carpal portion of the implant. Further implant development is needed to design implants with multiple metacarpal fixation stems to address this difficult problem. Until these implants are developed, custom implants may need to be used for these complex cases.

Future Research Needed

A paucity of literature exists on the topic of implant arthroplasty around the wrist when compared with hip and knee arthroplasty. The successes and failures of other joint replacements must be reviewed and understood. It will be important for all hand surgeons to share both favorable and unfavorable reports through publications so that continued development can be made in the right direction. Only with further scientific development will patients with arthritis around the wrist have improved outcomes in the future.

REFERENCES

1. Eaton RG, Lane LB, Littler JW, et al. Ligament reconstruction for the painful thumb carpometacarpal joint: a long-term assessment. J Hand Surg Am 1984;9:692–9.
2. Lane LB, Eaton RG. Ligament reconstruction for the painful "prearthritic" thumb carpometacarpal joint. Clin Orthop Relat Res 1987;220:52–7.
3. Freedman DM, Clickel SZ, Eaton RG. Long-term results of volar ligament reconstruction for symptomatic basal joint laxity. J Hand Surg Am 2000; 25:297–304.
4. Barron OA, Eaton RG. Save the trapezium: double interposition arthroplasty for the treatment of stage IV disease of the basal joint. J Hand Surg Am 1998; 23:196–204.
5. Tomaino MM. Basal Metacarpal Osteotomy for Osteoarthritis of the Thumb. J Hand Surg Am 2011;36:1076–9.
6. Parker WL, Linscheid RL, Amadio PC. Long-term outcomes of first metacarpal extension osteotomy in the treatment of carpal-metacarpal osteoarthritis. J Hand Surg Am 2008;33:1737–43.
7. Pellegrini VD Jr, Parentis M, Judkins A, et al. Extension metacarpal osteotomy in the treatment of trapeziometacarpal osteoarthritis: a biomechanical study. J Hand Surg Am 1996;21:16–23.
8. Martou G, Veltri K, Thoma A. Surgical treatment of osteoarthritis of the carpometacarpal joint of the thumb: a systematic review. Plast Reconstr Surg 2004;114:421–32.
9. Vermeulen GM, Slijper H, Feitz R, et al. Surgical management of primary thumb carpometacarpal osteoarthritis: a systematic review. J Hand Surg Am 2011;36:157–69.
10. Rizzo M, Moran SL, Shin AY. Long-term outcomes of trapeziometacarpal arthrodesis in the management of trapeziometacarpal arthritis. J Hand Surg Am 2009;34:20–6.
11. Gervis WH. Excision of the trapezium for osteoarthritis of the trapezio-metacarpal joint. J Bone Joint Surg Br 1949;31B(4):537–9.
12. Gervis WH, Wells T. A review of excision of the trapezium for osteoarthritis of the trapezio-metacarpal joint after twenty-five years. J Bone Joint Surg Br 1973;55:56–7.
13. Murley AH. Excision of the trapezium in osteoarthritis of the first carpometacarpal joint. J Bone Joint Surg Br 1960;42:502–7.
14. Swanson AB. Silicone rubber implants for replacement of arthritis or destroyed joints in the hand. Surg Clin North Am 1968;48:1113–27.
15. Minami A, Iwasaki N, Kutsumi K, et al. A long-term follow-up of silicone rubber interposition arthroplasty for osteoarthritis of the thumb carpometacarpal joint. Hand Surg 2005;10(1):77–82.
16. Nilsson A, Liljensten E, Bergström C, et al. Results from a degradable TMC joint Spacer (Artelon) compared with tendon arthroplasty. J Hand Surg 2005;30:380–9.
17. Jörheim M, Isaxon I, Flondell M, et al. Short-term outcomes of trapeziometacarpal Artelon implant compared with tendon suspension interposition arthroplasty for osteoarthritis: a matched cohort study. J Hand Surg Am 2009;34:1381–7.
18. Van Cappelle HG, Elzenga P, Van Horn JR. Long-term results and loosening analysis of de la Caffinière replacements of the trapeziometacarpal joint. J Hand Surg Am 1999;24(3):476–82.
19. Badia A, Sambandam SN. Total joint arthroplasty in the treatment of advanced stages of thumb carpometacarpal joint osteoarthritis. J Hand Surg Am 2006;31:1605.e1–1605.e13.
20. Ulrich-Vinther M, Puggaard H, Lange B. Prospective 1-year follow-up study comparing joint prosthesis with tendon interposition arthroplasty in treatment of trapeziometacarpal osteoarthritis. J Hand Surg Am 2008;33:1369–77.
21. Athwal GS, Chenkin J, King GJ, et al. Early failures with a spheric interposition arthroplasty of the thumb basal joint. J Hand Surg Am 2004;29: 1080–4.
22. Menon J. Partial trapeziectomy and interpositional arthroplasty for trapeziometacarpal osteoarthritis of the thumb. J Hand Surg Br 1995;20:700–6.
23. Burton RI, Pellegrini VD. Surgical management of basal joint arthritis of the thumb. Part II: ligament reconstruction with tendon interposition arthroplasty. J Hand Surg Am 1986;11:324–32.
24. Heyworth BE, Jobin CM, Monica JT, et al. Long-term follow-up of basal joint resection arthroplasty of the thumb with transfer of the abductor pollicis brevis origin to the flexor carpi radialis tendon. J Hand Surg Am 2009;34:1021–8.
25. Dhar S, Gray IC, Jones WA, et al. Simple excision of the trapezium for osteoarthritis of the carpometacarpal joint of the thumb. J Hand Surg Br 1994; 19(4):485–8.
26. Salem H, Davis TR. Six year outcome excision of the trapezium for trapeziometacarpal joint osteoarthritis: is it improved by ligament reconstruction and temporary Kirschner wire insertion? J Hand Surg Eur Vol 2012;37(3):211–9.

27. Edwards SG, Ramsey PN. Prospective outcomes of stage III thumb carpometacarpal arthritis treated with arthroscopic hemitrapeziectomy and thermal capsular modification without interposition. J Hand Surg Am 2010;35:566–71.

28. Davis TR, Brady O, Dias JJ. Excision of the trapezium for osteoarthritis of the trapeziometacarpal joint: a study of the benefit of ligament reconstruction or tendon interposition. J Hand Surg Am 2004; 29:1069–77.

29. Horlock N, Belcher HJ. Early versus late mobilisation after simple excision of the trapezium. J Bone Joint Surg Br 2002;84(8):1111–5.

30. Ely LW. An operation for tuberculosis of the wrist. JAMA 1920;75:1707–9.

31. Evans DL. Wedge arthrodesis of the wrist. J Bone Joint Surg Br 1955;37:126–34.

32. Larsson SE. Compression arthrodesis of the wrist: a consecutive series of 23 cases. Clin Orthop Relat Res 1974;99:146–53.

33. Mannerfelt L, Malmsten M. Arthrodesis of the wrist in rheumatoid arthritis: a technique without external fixation. Scand J Plast Reconstr Surg 1971;5: 124–30.

34. Wood MB. Wrist arthrodesis using dorsal radial bone graft. J Hand Surg Am 1987;12:208–12.

35. Peterson HA, Lipscomb PR. Intercarpal arthrodesis. Arch Surg 1967;95:127–34.

36. Watson JH, Hemptom RF. Limited wrist arthrodesis. I: the triscaphoid joint. J Hand Surg 1980;5:320–7.

37. Minamikawa Y, Peimer CA, Yamaguchi T, et al. Ideal scaphoid angle for intercarpal arthrodesis. J Hand Surg Am 1992;17:370–5.

38. Sutro CJ. Treatment of nonunion of the carpal navicular bone. Surgery 1946;20:536–40.

39. Helfet AJ. A new operation for ununited fractures of the scaphoid. J Bone Joint Surg Br 1952;34:329.

40. Pisano SM, Peimer CA, Wheeler DR, et al. Scaphocapitate intercarpal arthrodesis. J Hand Surg Am 1991;16:328–33.

41. Watson HK, Ballet FL. The SLAC wrist: scapholunate advanced collapse pattern of degenerative arthritis. J Hand Surg Am 1984;9:358–65.

42. Watson JH, Goodman ML, Johnson TR. Limited wrist arthrodesis. II: intercarpal and radial carpal combinations. J Hand Surg 1981;6:223–33.

43. Calandruccio JH, Gelberman RH, Duncan SF, et al. Capitolunate arthrodesis with scaphoid and triquetrum excision. J Hand Surg Am 2000;25:824–32.

44. Chamay A, Della Santa D, Vilaseca A. Radiolunate arthrodesis factor of stability for the rheumatoid wrist. Ann Chir Main 1983;2:5–17.

45. Elfar JC, Stern PJ. Proximal row carpectomy for scapholunate dissociation. J Hand Surg Br 2011; 36(2):111–5.

46. Mulford JS, Ceulemans LJ, Nam D, et al. Proximal row carpectomy vs four corner fusion for scapholunate (SLAC) or scaphoid nonunion advanced collapse (SNAC) wrists: a systematic review of outcomes. J Hand Surg Br 2009;34(2):256–63.

47. Richou J, Chuinard C, Moineau G, et al. Proximal row carpectomy: long-term results. Chir Main 2010;29(1):10–5.

48. McElfresh E. History of arthroplasty. In: Petty W, editor. Total joint replacement. Philadelphia: WB Saunders; 1991. p. 3–18.

49. Ritt MJ, Stuart PR, Naggar L, et al. The early history of arthroplasty of the wrist: from amputation to total wrist implant. J Hand Surg Br 1994;19(6):778–82.

50. Eynon-Lewis NJ, Ferry D, Pearse MF. Themistocles Gluck: an unrecognised genius. BMJ 1992;305: 1534–6.

51. Niebauer JJ, Landry RM. Dacron-Silicone. Prosthesis for the Metacarpophalangeal and Interphalangeal. J Hand Surg Eur Vol 1971;3(1):55–61.

52. Swanson AB. Flexible implant arthroplasty for arthritic disabilities of the radiocarpal joint: a silicone rubber intramedullary stemmed flexible hinge implant for the wrist joint. Orthop Clin North Am 1973;4(2):383–94.

53. Swanson AB, de Groot Swanson G. Flexible implant resection arthroplasty of the proximal interphalangeal joint. Hand Clin 1994;10(2):261–6.

54. Swanson AB. Implant resection arthroplasty of the proximal interphalangeal joint. Orthop Clin North Am 1973;4(4):1007–29.

55. Rossello MI, Costa M, Pizzorno V. Experience of total wrist arthroplasty with silastic implants plus grommets. Clin Orthop Relat Res 1997;342:64–70.

56. Fatti JF, Palmer AK, Mosher JF. The long-term results of Swanson silicone rubber interpositional wrist arthroplasty. J Hand Surg Am 1986;11(2): 166–75.

57. Fatti JF, Palmer AK, Greenky S, et al. Long-term results of Swanson interpositional wrist arthroplasty: Part II. J Hand Surg Am 1991;16:432–7.

58. Jolly SL, Ferlic DC, Clayton ML, et al. Swanson silicone arthroplasty of the wrist in rheumatoid arthritis: a long-term follow-up. J Hand Surg Am 1992;17:142–17149.

59. Meuli HC. Arthroplasty of the wrist. Clin Orthop Relat Res 1980;149:118–25.

60. Volz RG. Total wrist arthroplasty: a new approach to wrist disability. Clin Orthop 1977;128:180–9.

61. Volz RG. The development of a total wrist arthroplasty. Clin Orthop 1976;116:209–14.

62. Alnot J. L'Arthroplastie totale Guepar de poignet dona la polyarthrite rhumatoide. Acta Orthop Belg 1988;54(2):178–84.

63. Cooney WP, Beckenbaugh RD, Linscheid RL. Total wrist arthroplasty: problems with implant failures. Clin Orthop Relat Res 1984;187:121–8.

64. Cobb TK, Beckenbaugh RD. Biaxial total-wrist arthroplasty. J Hand Surg Am 1996;21:1011–21.

65. Talwalkar SC, Hayton MJ, Trail IA, et al. Management of the failed biaxial wrist replacement. J Hand Surg Br 2005;30(3):248–51.

66. Rizzo M, Beckenbaugh RD. Results of biaxial total wrist arthroplasty with a modified (long) metacarpal stem. J Hand Surg Am 2003;28(4):577–84.

67. Menon J. Universal total wrist implant. J Arthroplasty 1998;13:515–23.

68. Adams BD. Total wrist arthroplasty. Orthopedics 2004;27:278–84.

69. Gupta A. Total wrist arthroplasty. Am J Orthop 2008;37(8 Suppl 1):12–6.

70. Darrach W. Anterior dislocation of the head of the ulna. Ann Surg 1912;56:802–3.

71. Dingman PV. Resection of the distal end of the ulna (Darrach operation): an end result study of twenty four cases. J Bone Joint Surg Am 1952;34(4): 893–900.

72. Bowers WH. Distal radioulnar joint arthroplasty: the hemiresection-interposition technique. J Hand Surg Am 1985;10(2):169–78.

73. Watson HK, Ryu JY, Burgess RC. Matched distal ulnar resection. J Hand Surg Am 1986;11(6):812–7.

74. Sauvé L, Kapandji M. Nouvelle technique de traitement chirurgical des luxations récidivantes isolées de l'extrémité inférieure du cubitus. J Chirurgie (Paris) 1936;47:589–94.

75. Taleisnik J. The Sauvé-Kapandji procedure. Clin Orthop Relat Res 1992;275:110–23.

76. Milch H. Cuff resection of the ulna for malunited Colles' fracture. J Bone Joint Surg 1941;23:311–3.

77. Wehbé MA, Cautilli DA. Ulnar shortening using the AO small distractor. J Hand Surg Am 1995; 20:959–64.

78. Feldon P, Terrono AL, Belsky MR. Wafer distal ulna resection for triangular fibrocartilage tears and/or ulna impaction syndrome. J Hand Surg Am 1992; 17(4):731–7.

79. Adams BD, Berger RA. An anatomic reconstruction of the distal radioulnar ligaments for posttraumatic distal radioulnar joint instability. J Hand Surg Am 2002;27(2):243–51.

80. Swanson AB. Implant arthroplasty for disabilities of the distal radioulnar joint: Use of a silicone rubber capping implant following resection of the ulnar head. Orthop Clin North Am 1973;4(2):373–82.

81. Stanley D, Herbert TJ. The Swanson ulnar head prosthesis for post-traumatic disorders of the distal radio-ulnar joint. J Hand Surg Br 1992;17:682–8.

82. Wehbé MA. Pitfalls of radio-ulnar joint injuries. Philadelphia: Jefferson Orthopaedic Society Annual Meeting; November 15, 1991.

83. Scheker LR. Implant arthroplasty for the distal radioulnar joint. J Hand Surg Am 2008;33(9): 1639–44.

84. Schmalzried TP, Sahiri CA, Woolson ST. The significance of stem-cement loosening of grit-blasted femoral components. Orthopedics 2000;23(11): 1157–64.

85. Fini M, Giavaresi G, Torricelli P, et al. Osteoporosis and biomaterial osteointegration. Biomed Pharmacother 2004;58(9):487–93.

86. Hartman CW, Garvin KL. Femoral fixation in revision total hip arthroplasty. Instr Course Lect 2012; 61:313–25.

87. Bardou-Jacquet J, Souillac V, Mouton A, et al. Primary aseptic revision of the femoral component of a cemented total hip arthroplasty using a cemented technique without bone graft. Orthop Traumatol Surg Res 2009;95(4):243–8.

88. Lemons JE. Metallic alloys. In: Morrey B, editor. Joint replacement arthroplasty. 3rd edition. Philadelphia: Churchill-Livingstone; 1996. p. 19–27.

89. Bankston AB, Faris PM, Keating EM, et al. Polyethylene wear in total hip arthroplasty in patient matched groups. A comparison of stainless steel, cobalt chrome, and titanium-bearing surfaces. J Arthroplasty 1993;8(3):315–22.

90. Radmer S, Andresen R, Sparmann M. Total wrist arthroplasty in patients with rheumatoid arthritis. J Hand Surg Am 2003;28(5):789–94.

91. Long M, Rack HJ. Titanium alloys in total joint replacement—a materials science perspective. Biomaterials 1998;19(18):1621–39.

92. Daecke W, Veyel K, Weiloch P, et al. Osseointegration and mechanical stability of pyrocarbone and titanium hand implants in a load-bearing in vivo model for small joint arthroplasty. J Hand Surg Am 2006;31(1):90–7.

93. Jung M, Wieloch P, Lorenz H, et al. Comparison of cobalt chrome, ceramic and pyrocarbon hemiprosthesis in a rabbit model: ceramic leads to more cartilage damage than cobalt chromium. J Biomed Mater Res B Appl Biomater 2008;85(2): 427–34.

94. Wennerberg A, Albrektsson T. Effect of titanium surface topography on bone integration: a systematic review. Clin Oral Implants Res 2009;20(Suppl 4):172–84.

95. Jager M, Urselmann F, Witte F, et al. Osteoblast differentiation onto different biomaterials with an endoprosthetic surface topography in vitro. J Biomed Mater Res 2008;86(1):61–75.

96. Itala AI, Ylanen HO, Ekholm C, et al. Pore diameter of more than 100 microm is not a requisite for bone ingrowth in rabbits. J Biomed Mater Res 2001; 58(6):679–83.

97. Bobyn JD, Pilliar RM, Cameron HU, et al. The optimum pore size for the fixation of porous-surfaced metal implants by the ingrowth of bone. Clin Orthop Relat Res 1980;150:263–70.

98. Kienapfel H, Sprey C, Wilke A, et al. Implant fixation by bone ingrowth. J Arthroplasty 1999;14(3): 355–68.

99. Van Winterswijk PJ, Bakx PA. Promising clinical results of the universal total wrist prosthesis in rheumatoid arthritis. Open Orthop J 2010;4:67–70.

100. Ward CM, Kuhl T, Adams BD. Five to ten-year outcomes of the universal total wrist arthroplasty in patients with rheumatoid arthritis. J Bone Joint Surg Am 2011;93(10):914–9.

101. Lappalainen R, Santavirta SS. Potential of coatings in total hip replacement. Clin Orthop Relat Res 2005;430:72–9.

102. Schuurman AH, Teunis T. A new total distal radioulnar joint prosthesis: functional outcome. J Hand Surg Am 2010;35(10):1614–9.

103. Dimitriou R, Babis GC. Biomaterial osseointegration enhancement with biophysical stimulation. J Musculoskelet Neuronal Interact 2007;7(3):253–65.

104. Boyer JS, Adams B. Distal radius hemiarthroplasty combined with proximal row carpectomy: case report. Iowa Orthop J 2010;30:168–73.

105. Langton DJ, Jameson SS, Joyce TJ, et al. Accelerating failure rate of the ASR total hip replacement. J Bone Joint Surg Br 2011;93(8):1011–6.

106. Matthies AK, Skinner JA, Osmani H, et al. Pseudotumors are common in well-positioned low-wearing metal-on-metal hips. Clin Orthop Relat Res 2012; 470(7):1895–906.

107. O'Flynn HM, Roseen A, Weiland AJ. Failure of the hinge mechanism of a trispherical total wrist arthroplasty: a case report and review of the literature. J Hand Surg Am 1999;24(1):156–60.

108. Crisco JJ, Heard WM, Rich RR, et al. The mechanical axes of the wrist are oriented obliquely to the anatomic axes. J Bone Joint Surg Am 2011;93(2): 169–77.

109. Atwal NS, Clark DA, Amirfeyz R, et al. Salvage of a failed Suave-Kapandji procedure using a total distal radio-ulnar joint replacement. Hand Surg 2010;15(2):119–22.

110. Dunbar MJ, Richardson G. Minimizing infection risk: fortune favors the prepared mind. Orthopedics 2011;34(9):467–9.

111. Scanzello CR, Figgie MP, Nestor BJ, et al. Perioperative management of medications used in the treatment of rheumatoid arthritis. HSS J 2006; 2(2):141–7.

112. Mater WY, Jafari SM, Restrepo C, et al. Preventing infection in total joint arthroplasty. J Bone Joint Surg Am 2010;92(Suppl 2):36–46.

113. Della Valle C, Parvizi J, Bauer TW, et al. American Academy of Orthopaedic Surgeons clinical practice guidelines on: the diagnosis of periprosthetic joint infections of the hip and knee. J Bone Joint Surg Am 2011;93(14):1355–7.

114. Rizzo M, Ackerman DB, Rodrigues RL, et al. Wrist arthrodesis as a salvage procedure for failed implant arthroplasty. J Hand Surg Eur Vol 2011;36(1):29–33.

115. Carlson JR, Simmons BP. Wrist arthrodesis after failed wrist implant arthroplasty. J Hand Surg Am 1998;23(5):893–8.

116. Chin KR, Spak JI, Jupiter JB. Septic arthritis and osteomyelitis of the wrist: reconstruction with a vascularized fibular graft. J Hand Surg Am 1999;24(2): 243–8.

117. Frigg A, Dougall H, Boyd S. Can porous tantalum be used to achieve ankle and subtalar arthrodesis?: a pilot study. Clin Orthop Relat Res 2010;468(1): 209–16.

118. Cobb TK, Beckenbaugh RD. Biaxial long-stemmed multipronged distal components for revision/bone deficit total-wrist arthroplasty. J Hand Surg Am 1996;21(5):764–70.

Ligament Reconstruction and Tendon Interposition for Thumb Basal Arthritis

John C. Elfar, MD*, Richard I. Burton, MD

KEYWORDS

- Basal joint arthritis • Carpometacarpal joint of thumb
- Ligament reconstruction and tendon interposition • Basal joint arthroplasty

KEY POINTS

- Arthritis at the base of the thumb is common and debilitating. Arthroplasty has evolved over three decades to become a highly refined surgical procedure, with excellent results.
- After summarizing the history, method, and expected results of basal joint arthroplasty, the authors describe their method of ligament reconstruction and tendon interposition for thumb basal arthritis.
- The goal of successful treatment of thumb basal joint arthritis is relief of pain with retention of motion and stability.

INTRODUCTION

The goal of successful treatment of thumb basal joint arthritis is relief of pain with retention of motion and stability. Fusion by various techniques[1,2] achieves relief of pain but at the cost of lost motion. Since 1947,[3] arthritis of the thumb has been treated with various types of arthroplasty in an attempt to relieve pain and preserve motion, but often with resulting instability and/or weakness. Arthroplasties involving implants have been associated with various problems including particulate synovitis, subsidence, and/or dislocation.

Arthroplasty for the base of the thumb has gone through many refinements over the years. In the past, advanced disease at the carpometacarpal (CMC) joint of the thumb at presentation was the rule. Tackling this disease necessitated the development of techniques that allowed for the treatment of a wide array of problems. The treatment options evolved to deal with various stages of the disease.

There is no consensus on the critical elements of arthroplasty for the base of the thumb, as surgeons seem to rely mostly on their experience to pursue critical elements and variations in arthroplasty technique to ensure a pain-free and strong thumb long after surgery.

HISTORY

The ideal arthroplasty relieves pain, provides stability, and retains or improves strength. Arthroplasty pursues one of two general schemes. The first is to resurface the opposing joint surfaces with artificial noninnervated alternatives; the second is to resect the joint surfaces and to reconstruct attenuated or missing ligaments, and interpose material or tissue in between the bone ends. These arthroplasty methods contrast with simple resection of the joint as seen in trapeziectomy, or fusion, both of which are classic treatments for painful CMC joint arthritis.[1–3]

The evolution of resection and interpositional arthroplasty has led to surgical principles that underlie a variety of surgical procedures. Some of the concepts in the surgical treatment of basal joint

The authors have nothing to disclose for this work.

Department of Orthopaedics, School of Medicine and Dentistry, University of Rochester Medical Center, Rochester, NY, USA

* Corresponding author. Department of Orthopaedics, University of Rochester, 601 Elmwood Avenue, Box 665, Rochester, NY 14642.

E-mail address: openelfar@gmail.com

osteoarthritis originate from the treatment of inflammatory rheumatoid arthritis (RA) in the era before disease-modifying antirheumatic drugs. In that setting, with the long-term shortcomings of silicone arthroplasty still unknown, many RA patients had very successful implant arthroplasty for basal joint arthritis. These procedures were based on the principle that a soft artificial spacer that maintained the distance between painful bone ends could decrease pain by interposing noninnervated material while retaining strength because of maintained thumb length. In this way, implant arthroplasty was preferable to arthrodesis, which offers pain relief in exchange for motion.

Unfortunately, the success with silicone basal joint arthroplasty for the rheumatoid patient did not prove to be the situation with the higher demand hand seen in osteoarthritis. Over the decades between the introduction of the silicone arthroplasty for basal joint in RA and its large-scale abandonment in the treatment of osteoarthritis of the basal joint, the consequences of silicone interposition in small joints began to appear: (1) fragmentation, (2) instability, (3) particulate synovitis, and (4) cold flow deformation.[4] Failure of silicone interposition arthroplasty when applied to the osteoarthritic thumb basal joint often led to revision surgery whereby salvage fusion was either difficult or impossible to achieve in the setting of a foreign-body reaction and decreased bone stock. The failure of a reliable interposition using foreign materials fueled the search for a reliable biological interpositional and stabilizing procedure free from the problems seen with the prosthetic implants.

At the same time, there evolved a nuanced understanding of the pathophysiology of basal joint osteoarthritis. At its earliest stage, shear forces at the trapeziometacarpal joint cause subluxation of the joint and incompetency of the palmar oblique ligament. Ligamentous reconstruction in early-stage, unstable trapeziometacarpal joint was also meeting with success regarding prevention of instability and subluxation.[5,6]

It was the combination of these 2 seemingly separate treatments, (1) ligament reconstruction for early instability with (2) biological interposition, which led to successful treatment of basal joint arthritis without foreign material. This approach combined the stabilizing effect of the ligament reconstruction with the standard arthroplasty principles of interposition with autologous tissue.[7–9]

Since the development of this combined approach, much has evolved both in the presurgical treatment and surgical variations on treatment. Some surgical treatments exclude one or another portion of the technique described herein in an effort to distill the minimal, critical elements of surgical treatment. What follows is a description of the authors' surgical technique, which aims to provide a single reliable basal joint arthroplasty procedure that can be applied to a wide range of pathologic states in this joint.

INDICATIONS FOR LIGAMENT RECONSTRUCTION WITH TENDON INTERPOSITION

Ligament reconstruction with tendon interposition was first introduced in the 1970s in the population of patients older than 50 years with very symptomatic and severe basal joint arthritis.[8,10] However, in the decades since the introduction of this procedure, the indications have extended to younger age groups.[11,12]

Mild cases of basal joint arthritis with relative preservation of the joint can be treated with other procedures such as the Eaton ligament reconstruction,[5] metacarpal extension osteotomy,[13] and more recently, carpometacarpal arthroscopic debridement.[14,15] Alternatively, if basal joint arthroplasty is not an option because of high demands placed as part of athletic or work-related needs, arthrodesis is still the treatment of choice with the preferred technique described by Eaton and Littler.[1] One particularly attractive advantage of fusion with the Eaton-Littler technique is the relative ease with which it can be revised to a tendon interposition with ligament reconstruction, should the need arise, because of subsequent scaphotrapeziotrapezoidal arthritis or symptoms at the thumb metacarpophalangeal (MP) joint.

PREOPERATIVE CONSIDERATIONS AND COEXISTING CONDITIONS

Multiple conditions may coexist with basal joint arthritis, including DeQuervain tenosynovitis[16] and carpal tunnel syndrome.[17] A careful history and physical examination can often reveal if either of these conditions contributes to pain on the radial side of the wrist and weakness in the thenar musculature. The existence of these conditions should be considered in formulating an operative plan for the patient who has failed nonoperative treatment.

Preoperatively, the evaluation should also assess the MP joint of the thumb. If more than 30° of MP extension or valgus instability is found, the operative plan should also address this instability. The standard approach to such a patient includes arthrodesis of the MP joint in 15° to 20° of flexion, with 15° to 20° of pronation, or one of a variety of soft-tissue procedures.

TECHNIQUE
Anesthesia

The preferred form of anesthetic is the regional axillary block. Advantages include continued postoperative pain relief in addition to safety. Patients typically awaken from sedation without postoperative nausea and are able to return home shortly after the procedure.

Incision

Many approaches have been used to successfully expose the trapeziometacarpal joint.[18,19] Although the anterior and anterolateral approaches have led to successful results, the posterolateral triradiate approach described here allows for concomitant surgical treatment of the common copresenting DeQuervain tenosynovitis. The senior author has used the posterolateral triradiate approach to perform thousands of basal joint arthroplasty procedures.

For this approach, anatomic observations can be used to very accurately define the preferred location of the incision. When the patient is anesthetized, the basal joint grind test is used to mark the exact location of the CMC joint on the radial surface of the hand. The radial artery is palpated as it traverses the anatomic snuffbox and accurately locates the scaphotrapezial (ST) joint. With these landmarks (Fig. 1A), a longitudinal incision is made along the proximal shaft of the metacarpal and is continued to the level of the ST joint, at which point 2 separate limbs of the triradiate incision are extended in palmar and dorsal proximal directions. One planned incision will be made later in the procedure to harvest the entire proximal flexor carpi radialis (FCR) tendon (Fig. 1B).

During dissection, multiple branches of the radial sensory nerve are encountered and must be protected (Fig. 1C). Experience has taught that these nerves are best left in their protective fatty envelope of soft tissue and not finely skeletonized. These nerve branches are protected by gentle retraction with moistened Ragnell retractors (self-retaining retractors are never used here). Later, the placement of capsular sutures will allow the gentle retraction of these deep soft-tissue flaps, which hold these delicate nerves out of the way.

Radial Artery

The radial artery resides in the interval between the extensor pollicis brevis (EPB) and abductor pollicis longus (APL) tendons, as it courses from palmar to dorsal. It is this distal route that brings it closest to the deep ulnar beak of the trapezium as the artery enters into the first web space. The artery is mobilized away from the ST joint and distal scaphoid, and carefully retracted, with care taken to coagulate small branches of the artery located at the ST joint in the anatomic snuffbox (Fig. 2).

Trapezial Excision

Beneath the former position of the radial artery is the capsule of the ST joint. The capsule of the CMC joint, the periosteum of the trapezium, and the ST capsule are incised longitudinally, with care taken to ensure the further trapezial dissection remains subperiosteal in the palmar and

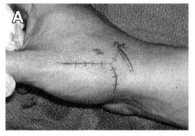
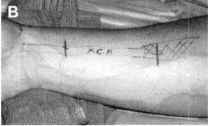
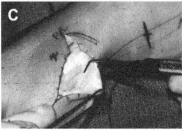

Fig. 1. (A) Putative plan for incision for main surgical procedure. (B) Plan for flexor carpi radialis (FCR) harvest. (C) Note the branch of the radial sensory nerve.

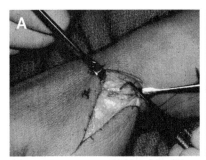
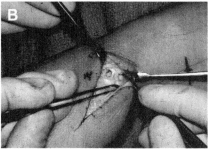

Fig. 2. (*A*) Native position of radial artery. (*B*) Mobilized and proximally displaced artery revealing the capsule of the carpometacarpal joint.

dorsal directions. This action ensures safety to the dorsal structures already mentioned in addition to the thenar muscles and FCR in the deep portion of the wound. The landmarks for the dissection are the dorsal extent of the trapeziotrapezoid (TT) joint and palmar extent of the trapezium to the ridge overlying the FCR, well beneath the thenar muscles. At this point, capsular sutures are placed to facilitate later repair of the capsule. Gentle traction on these sutures allows the protection of the radial sensory nerves as already noted. Once this has been done, small Homan retractors are placed: 1 palmar, 1 dorsal, and 1 in the ST. The trapezium is now fully visualized and isolated (**Fig. 3**).

The trapezium is then scored with a sagittal saw to 75% depth of the trapezial bone in cruciate configuration so as to ensure safety to the FCR tendon, which courses deep to the bone (**Fig. 3**). It is important to orient the longitudinal cut parallel to the course of the FCR tendon so as to decrease the likelihood of tendon injury should the cut be inadvertently made too deep. An osteotome is used to lever in the saw cuts using a twisting motion which "pops" the trapezium into 4 pieces, and the bone is removed in 4 quadrants. An effort is made to ensure complete excision of

the trapezium from the valley occupied by the medial beak of the bone. Large and small osteophytes and loose bodies are removed at this time. Special attention should be paid to the deep cul-de-sac at the beak of the metacarpal between the base of the first and second metacarpals. This area often harbors loose bodies hidden from view.

Preparation for the Ligament Reconstruction

Subperiosteal dissection is done along the base of the metacarpal to a level 1 cm distal to the metacarpal base; this will be the planned exit point of the new ligament reconstruction. The entry point will be on the deep side of the metacarpal base at the former attachment site of the old palmarbeak ligament. A channel through the proximal metacarpal bone will have to connect these 2 points. The channel is created with gouges and curettes, with appropriate retraction to protect the extensor tendon and sensory nerves (**Fig. 4**).

Flexor Carpi Radialis Harvest

The FCR is now visualized in the defect left by the trapezial excision. Dissection and slight tension on it in this space can free it from scarring often seen at the distal scaphoid and attachment to the palmar and deep capsule. It must be freed to the level of its insertion on the second metacarpal.

The musculotendinous junction of the FCR is next identified by palpation through intact skin in the mid-proximal forearm. A single transverse incision is made over this site with dissection to the level of the deep fascia. The tendon is identified and a curved hemostat is passed beneath the tendon. The tendon is transected, and adjacent muscle fibers (usually deep to the tendon) need to be sharply freed from the tendon.

Traction is then placed either with a dental probe, or umbilical tape preplaced around the tendon in the arthroplasty space, and the tendon

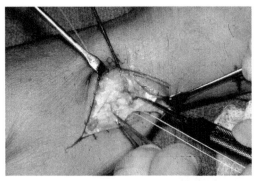

Fig. 3. Retention sutures hold the capsule open and allow for later tight closure over the interposition bolus.

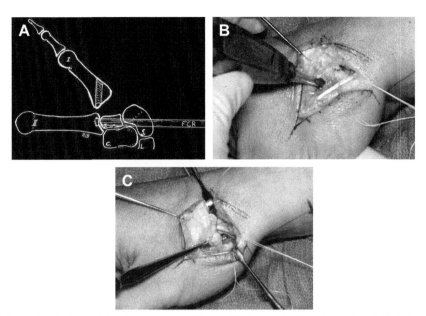

Fig. 4. (*A*) Schematic of channel in the metacarpal base. (*B*) Gouge in the channel as it is being formed. (*C*) Completed channel.

is delivered into the distal wound. If difficulty is encountered delivering the free end of the tendon, a second transverse incision may be needed just proximal to the wrist midway between the 2 incisions (**Fig. 5**). This tendon is then wrapped in a moistened gauze sponge.

Extraneous muscle fibers are removed sharply from the tendon, and a deep number-2 Ethibond suture (Ethicon, Cornelia, GA) on a small needle is placed in the FCR just proximal to its insertion on the second metacarpal at the deepest portion of the arthroplasty space. This suture is placed so that it can be used to secure the FCR tendon deep in the arthroplasty space after the tendon is passed through the metacarpal base boney channel. At this point, the tendon is passed through the channel and allowed to exit the dorsal side of the metacarpal. This passage of the tendon through the bone tunnel is facilitated by tightly tying a 26-gauge wire 2 mm from the cut end of the FCR, passing the 2 ends of this wire from deep to

superficial through the tunnel, and then gently delivering the tendon through the tunnel; a soft circular motion with the gentle traction is often helpful.

In the arthroplasty space, the deep capsule is repaired at its depth with at least 2 sutures of 3-0 or 4-0 monofilament nonabsorbable sutures. The needle is removed from the suture, but the tails of each are left long and separately clamped for the subsequent placement of the interposition, as shown in **Fig. 6**. In addition to these 2 sutures, multiple additional sutures are often necessary for the deep capsular closure. Because of the small deep space that must accept these sutures, small curved needles are useful for the completion of this very important careful deep capsular repair and the placement of the retention sutures. This deep capsular closure, combined with the very tight lateral/superficial capsular closure done after the interposition, ensures the interposition is securely enclosed.

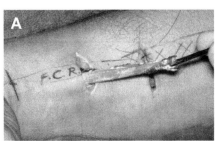
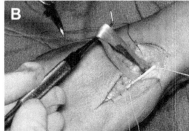

Fig. 5. (*A*) Harvest of the FCR. (*B*) Passing of FCR into the arthroplasty space.

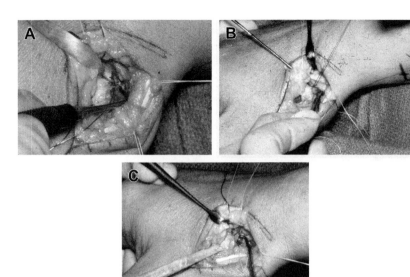

Fig. 6. (*A*) The deep capsule is closed and (*B*) sutures are kept long, emanating from the deep closure to allow for insertion of the interpositional bolus. (*C*) The FCR is passed through the channel.

Thumb Positioning and Kirschner-Wire Placement

It is essential that the position of the thumb in space, and therefore the size and position of the arthroplasty, is precise. If the projection of the thumb metacarpal from the fixed unit is the same as would be used for a CMC fusion, the maximum of thumb function will occur with the least amount of displacement force on the reconstruction. The following elements should guide the placement of the thumb relative to the fixed unit: (1) the thumb projection should be coaxial with the scaphoid; (2) the thumb metacarpal must project from the fixed unit in the fist position such that the thumb tip rests over the middle phalanx of the index finger with the thumb placed in the fist position; (3) 1 to 2 mm of space should be maintained between the base of the first and second metacarpals; and (4) the base of the thumb metacarpal should be at the same level as the base of the index metacarpal, thereby ensuring no overdistraction or underdistraction of the thumb arthroplasty space.

For these reasons, 1 or 2 Kirschner (K) pins are placed to hold the thumb metacarpal in this proper position relative to the fixed unit. The K-wire(s) must not traverse the boney tunnel or the arthroplasty space, as this would preclude proper tension on the ligament and/or proper placement of the interposition material (**Fig. 7**A, B). The K-wire will also serve to limit compression of the interpositional arthroplasty under the weight of the dressing and splint in the early postoperative period. With the thumb metacarpal properly positioned and

stabilized in this manner, maximum function is ensured with the least stress on the new "ligament." Firm traction is applied to the FCR tendon, so "it's as tight as it will go," with the metacarpal secure in the exact position desired. A stay suture is used to secure the tendon at the exit hole of the channel from the metacarpal bone (**Fig. 7**C). This stay suture goes from the dorsal metacarpal periosteum at the level of the exit hole in the bone, through the FCR, through the volar metacarpal periosteum, and thence back through the FCR and the dorsal periosteum. It should be placed with simultaneous gentle proximal traction on the capsular sutures to the maximum capsule for adequate lateral closure later.

The metacarpal base is resurfaced to completely cover the hole in the metacarpal base left by making the channel. This action eliminates the possibility of the interposition bolus from migrating into the metacarpal base itself. The FCR is folded back on itself. After ensuring that the tendon is draped across the surface of the metacarpal base, the tendon is sutured to itself in the depth of the arthroplasty space with the preplaced suture in the FCR, where it inserts into the second metacarpal base (**Fig. 8**A).

Interposition

The interposition tendon material should have the characteristics of a firm cushion of appropriate size.

Approximately 3 inches (7.6 cm) of FCR tendon are usually available for the interposition. A Keith

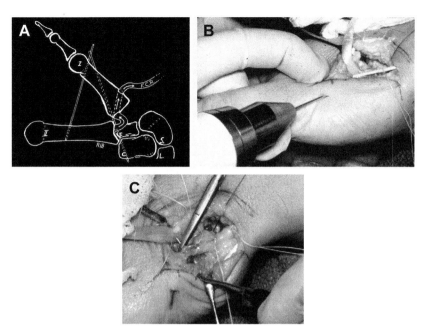

Fig. 7. (*A*) Schematic depicting the plan of placement of K-wires with the thumb in the functional position. (*B*) K-wire placement. (*C*) Suture of the snugly tensioned tendon to periosteal tissue.

needle is passed through the FCR tendon at the level of the skin. Successive 1-cm lengths of the remaining tendon are folded over the needle to form an interposition, which resembles a neatly folded ribbon candy (**Fig. 8**B). It normally takes 8 to 10 such folds to completely fold the FCR tendon in the form of an accordion (**Fig. 8**C).

At this point, a second Keith needle is passed through the bolus parallel to the first, and the needles are advanced through the bolus to compress

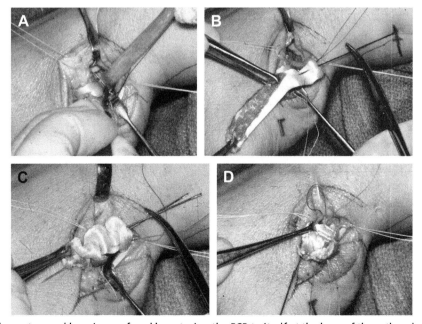

Fig. 8. (*A*) The metacarpal base is resurfaced by suturing the FCR to itself at the base of the arthroplasty space. (*B*) The interpositional bolus is formed by folding the tendon over a Keith needle. (*C*) The tendon is fully folded in the form of an accordion. (*D*) The quadrants of the tendon interposition are sutured and the needles threaded, with the deep sutures passed across the bolus.

the interposition. Sutures are then placed in each of the 4 quadrants of the interposition to firmly hold the tendon in this configuration. The Keith needles are then threaded with the previously placed sutures from the deep capsular closure so that further advancement of the Keith needles threads these sutures onto the bolus (**Fig. 8**D). Gentle traction is then placed on the flaps of the superficial capsule to create an open "funnel" into the arthroplasty space, and the bolus of interpositional tendon is then advanced into that space. The sutures threaded through the bolus are then tied to each other to hold the interposition firm to the base of the arthroplasty space. At this point, the configuration of the sutures and the bolus should ensure that (1) the bolus is pulled tightly into the trapezial space and (2) the bolus is stable (**Fig. 9**A, B).

Closure

The capsule is closed with the preplaced sutures used to open the arthroplasty space and allow the bolus to be inserted. If these lateral capsular structures do not include a firm attachment to the distal scaphoid, a fine K-wire is used to place a drill hole in the distal scaphoid through which 1 or 2 additional capsular closure sutures may be placed. Care is taken to ensure that the tight capsular closure is free of gaps and defects, usually accomplished by tying sutures in opposite flaps of the capsule together in a directly side-to-side configuration.

Transfer of the Extensor Pollicis Brevis

If the MP joint is not fused, a transfer of EPB can serve to decrease the extension force on the MP and increase the abduction power of the metacarpal away from the fixed unit. This transfer is accomplished by first suturing the EPB over the FCR tendon, which exits the bone channel, and then transecting the EPB distal to this point over the metacarpal (**Fig. 10**A, B). The remaining EPB is then tucked into the channel itself so as to recreate a tendon-to-bone interface when it has healed (**Fig. 10**C). The opening of the channel is then closed with a 4-0 purse-string nonabsorbable monofilament suture.

Pins are cut 2 to 3 mm superficial to the skin to allow easy removal in the office, and the wound is closed with fine nylon suture with care taken to avoid any branches of the radial sensory nerve in the closure. The skin-to-pin interface is coated with collodion in 2 or 3 applications.

DRESSING AND POSTOPERATIVE CARE
First Month

The position of the wrist in the postoperative dressing is important to the final result. Care is taken to position the wrist in approximately 15° to 25° of extension and in neutral radial-ulnar

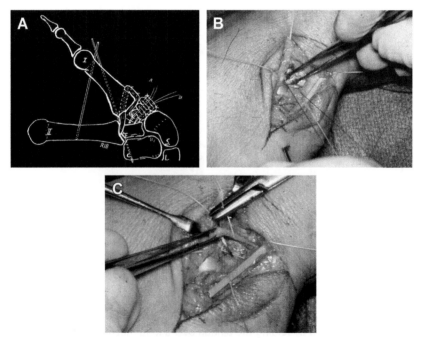

Fig. 9. (*A*) Schematic depicting inserted interpositional bolus with sutures in deep capsule. (*B*) Bolus inserted into arthroplasty space. (*C*) Tight capsular closure over bolus.

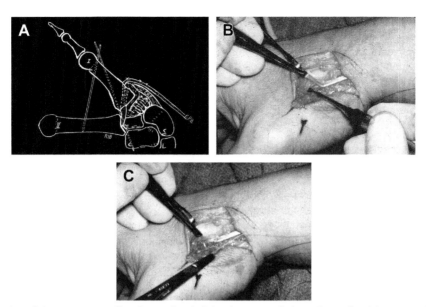

Fig. 10. Transfer of the extensor pollicis brevis (EPB). (*A*) Schematic of plan of transfer. (*B*) Suture of EPB to FCR exiting the channel. (*C*) Tucking and closing of the channel over the transfer of EPB.

deviation. Some extension is necessary so that the weight of the dressing and plaster shell while the hand is elevated is borne by the palm and pin and not the thumb; this helps to minimize the postoperative pain. Excessive wrist extension potentially compromises the ability to engage in rehabilitation exercises to achieve active wrist flexion, because of the lack of an active FCR muscle and immobilization in extension for 4 weeks.

Patients can be transferred to a cast at 1 week or can remain in the postoperative splint for an entire month. During the first month, the hand is kept elevated at all times, and the use of a foam wrist elevation pillow or similar device is helpful. Slings are avoided for their dependent positioning of the hand and the immobilization of the shoulder, which can lead to stiffness. Should discomfort arise after 1 or 2 weeks owing to decreased swelling and increased movement in the dressing, the dressing is changed and sutures removed, and a short-arm thumb spica cast is applied for the remainder of the first month after surgery. During the first month, finger range of motion along with range of motion of the thumb interphalangeal (IP) joint is encouraged with a home program several times per day.

Second Month

At 4 weeks, the K-wires are removed along with sutures. The patient is fitted with a forearm-based thumb spica splint. This phase emphasizes range of motion in the entire upper extremity with a focus on flexion and extension of the wrist and thenar muscle isometric strengthening, especially opponens muscle setting, as this muscle with its fibers nearly perpendicular to the metacarpal is especially important for stability of the metacarpal base. Specific elements of the wrist program include forearm wrist and hand being placed on a flat surface in supination with the wrist in 25° to 30° of extension, emphasizing controlled active wrist flexion from 30° of extension through a flexion arc of 45° to 50°.

Three to 6 Months

After 2 months, there is a gradual return to functional use in the activities of daily living. At 2 to 3 months the patient is weaned out of the splint, starting with gentle activities such a daily hygiene, eating, and writing. There is a gradual transition to unprotected full activity. Wrist weights are increased gradually to 6 lb (2.7 kg) and the repetitions are increased. Gripping, pinching, and pulling putty are added to the regimen after about 2 months along with manipulation of clothespins. All of the gripping exercises are performed with the thumb metacarpal in the position of functional activity (thumb positioned between palmar and radial abduction with IP joint free). No attempts are made to pinch to the ring or small fingers, as these motions risk stretching out the ligament reconstruction and have no functional use in activities of daily living. For the same reason, stretching the thumb into the palm-flat position is avoided.

Timing for return to work depends on the occupational manual needs and whether or not the dominant hand is the one operated on. Some executive positions permit return to work within a week. Higher-demand manual situations may require 3 to 6 months before a return to work, depending on the hand involved and rapidity in regaining excellent strength with the exercise program. Therapy exercises are continued for 1 to 2 years postoperatively; these are simple putty exercises that the patient does on his or her own.

Beyond 6 Months

The patient is encouraged to continue using the putty for an indefinite period after the surgery (6 to 36 months postoperatively). When these procedures were first done in the 1970s, the physicians and therapists assumed that maximum strength and function would occur within 3 to 6 months. To the pleasant surprise of all, patients continued to gain in strength for up to 1 to 2 years. Patients with a return of symptoms can reliably be found to have weakness attributable to discontinuation of exercises. Simple resumption of the strengthening program resolves these symptoms.

RESULTS

Although multiple procedures have been described for basal joint arthritis, the heterogeneity of procedures performed prevents the valid comparisons across different surgical series. Multiple studies have documented the short-, medium-, and long-term results of basal joint arthroplasty procedures.[12,20] The technique described here has led to very good patient satisfaction and high objective measures of function, including return of strength and dexterity to even the severely affected thumb.[12]

In the longest-term study to date of the procedure described in this article, Tomaino and colleagues[12] examined 24 thumbs of 22 patients at an average of 9 years (range, 8–11 years) after a ligament reconstruction–tendon interposition arthroplasty for osteoarthritis at the base of the thumb. The data included preoperative and sequential long-term follow-up on the same cohort of patients. The same cohort of patients had been followed previous to this longer-term follow-up at 2 and 6 years postoperatively. Three of the thumbs were revisions of failed implant arthroplasty, and the rest were performed as primary procedures.

Of this cohort, 21 (95%) were satisfied and had excellent pain relief. Objective improvement in grip strength was 10 kg-force (93% improvement) and tip pinch strength of nearly 2.2 lb (1 kg) (65% improvement). Key-pinch improvement was more modest, with 34% gain over preoperative values. Range of motion of the thumb tip returned to

flexion to the base of the small finger in 92% of patients with an average first web angle of 40°.

Stress radiographs showed an average subluxation of the metacarpal base of 11% at 9 years compared with 7% and 8% at 2 and 6 years, respectively. Similarly, these radiographs demonstrated an average loss of height of the arthroplasty space of 13% at 9 years compared with 11% at both of the earlier follow-up examinations. None of the modest changes in radiographic outcome predicted unsatisfactory outcome.

Taken together, these results were interpreted to suggest that the procedure described here led to a stable and functional reconstruction of the thumb, resulting in excellent relief of pain and a significant increase in strength for as long as 11 years after the procedure.[12]

SUMMARY

The frequency of occurrence and the significant symptoms with functional impairment from basal joint arthritis has motivated many advances in surgical procedures for this condition. Basal joint arthroplasty with ligament reconstruction and tendon interposition is the authors' treatment of choice, and can lead to reliable results in a variety of situations. It is this reliability, in the face of many variations of arthritis of the thumb, which has led to the popularity of ligament reconstruction and tendon interposition arthroplasty. The procedure is somewhat tedious to execute correctly with all its components being key to a successful outcome. However, the conscientious attention to detail of the surgical procedure as described herein leads to excellent long-term results.

REFERENCES

1. Eaton RG, Littler JW. A study of the basilar joint of the thumb. Treatment of its disabilities by fusion. J Bone Joint Surg Am 1969;51:661–8.
2. Carroll RE, Hill NA. Arthrodesis of the carpometacarpal joint of the thumb. J Bone Joint Surg Br 1973;55:292–4.
3. Gervis WH. Excision of the trapezium for osteoarthritis of the trapezio-metacarpal joint. J Bone Joint Surg Br 1949;31:537–9.
4. Pellegrini VD Jr, Burton RI. Surgical management of basilar joint arthritis of the thumb. Part I. Long-term results of silicone implant arthroplasty and Part II. Ligament reconstruction with tendon interposition arthroplasty. J Hand Surg Am 1986;11:309–24, 324–32.
5. Eaton RG, Lane LB, Littler JW, et al. Ligament reconstruction for the painful thumb carpometacarpal

joint: a long-term assessment. J Hand Surg Am 1984;9:692–9.

6. Glickel SZ, Malerich M, Pearce SM, et al. Ligament replacement for chronic instability of the ulnar collateral ligament of the metacarpophalangeal joint of the thumb. J Hand Surg Am 1993;18:930–41.

7. Uriburu IJ, Olazábal AE, Ciaffi M. Trapeziometacarpal osteoarthritis: surgical technique and results of "stabilized resection-arthroplasty". J Hand Surg Am 1992;17:598–604.

8. Burton RI. The arthritic hand: arthritis of the basilar joint. In: McCollister Evarts C, Burton RI, editors. Surgery of the musculoskeletal system. New York: Churchill Livingstone; 1983.

9. Thompson JS. Surgical treatment of trapeziometacarpal arthrosis. Adv Orthop Surg 1986;10:105–20.

10. Burton RI. Ligament reconstruction by tendon transfer and soft tissue interposition arthroplasty for basilar joint osteoarthritis of the thumb. (LRTI or Burton procedure). In: Master techniques in orthopaedic surgery: the hand. Philadelphia: Lippincott-Raven; 1998.

11. Burton RI, Pellegrini VD Jr. Basilar joint arthritis of thumb. J Hand Surg Am 1987;12:645.

12. Tomaino MM, Pellegrini VD Jr, Burton RI. Arthroplasty of the basilar joint of the thumb. Long-term follow-up after ligament reconstruction with tendon interposition. J Bone Joint Surg Am 1995;77:346–55.

13. Uzumcugil A. Long-term outcomes of first metacarpal extension osteotomy in the treatment of carpometacarpal osteoarthritis. J Hand Surg Am 2009;34:1156 [author reply: 1156–7].

14. Kapoutsis DV, Dardas A, Day CS. Carpometacarpal and scaphotrapeziotrapezoid arthritis: arthroscopy, arthroplasty, and arthrodesis. J Hand Surg Am 2011;36:354–66.

15. Yao J, Park MJ. Early treatment of degenerative arthritis of the thumb carpometacarpal joint. Hand Clin 2008;24:251–61, v–vi.

16. Burton RI. Complications following surgery on the basilar joint of the thumb. Hand Clin 1986;2: 265–9.

17. Florack TM, Miller RJ, Pellegrini VD, et al. The prevalence of carpal tunnel syndrome in patients with basilar joint arthritis of the thumb. J Hand Surg Am 1992;17:624–30.

18. Cassidy C, Glennon PE, Stein AB, et al. Basilar joint arthroplasty and carpal tunnel release through a single incision: an in vitro study. J Hand Surg Am 2004;29:1085–8.

19. Wagner CJ. Method of treatment of Bennett's fracture dislocation. Am J Surg 1950;80:230–1.

20. Kochevar AJ, Adham CN, Adham MN, et al. Thumb basilar joint arthroplasty using abductor pollicis longus tendon: an average 5.5-year follow-up. J Hand Surg Am 2011;36:1326–32.

Trapezium Resection with Mersilene Suspension Sling

Marwan A. Wehbé, MD[a,b,*], Rita M. Ciccarello, RN[a],
Jennifer L. Reitz, OTR/L, CHT[c]

KEYWORDS

- Trapezium - Arthroplasty - Trapeziectomy - Trapezoidectomy - Mersilene - Polyester
- Suspension - STT joint - LRTI

KEY POINTS

- Thumb carpometacarpal (CMC) joint arthrosis is one of the most common degenerative diseases that hand surgeons see.
- In this article, arthritis, arthrosis, and degenerative joint disease (DJD) will be used interchangeably.
- If a patient is lucky as was one of the authors' mentors, a notable orthopedic surgeon, the CMC joint may become ankylosed and pain could abate. Otherwise, the numerous available treatments for thumb CMC arthritis serve only to postpone the inexorable surgery.

Thumb carpometacarpal (CMC) joint arthrosis is one of the most common degenerative diseases that hand surgeons see. In this article, arthritis, arthrosis, and degenerative joint disease are used interchangeably. Otherwise, the numerous available treatments for thumb CMC arthritis serve only to postpone the inexorable surgery. Medication, steroid injections, splints, osteotomies, and "minimalist" surgeries do not seem to provide long-term relief for this potentially debilitating disorder. The scaphotrapeziotrapezoid (STT) joint is often involved, and a trapeziectomy with partial trapezoidectomy may be the only option that would alleviate pain and restore function.

Many of the numerous procedures designed to treat thumb basilar joint surgery are described in detail elsewhere in this book. The old standard that everyone is trying to beat is simple resection of the trapezium with no interposition of any kind

and no ancillary measures. The reason we are all trying to improve on that procedure is the proximal migration of the first metacarpal, with ensuing painful impingement on the distal scaphoid. This has been termed thumb subsidence or shortening. It follows that if we can prevent subsidence, we may prevent recurrence of the pain. Approaches to this problem consist of soft tissue procedures or prosthetic interposition. The authors present here what they believe to be the least mutilating of such procedures.

MERSILENE SUSPENSION SLING

Mersilene is a nonabsorbable woven polyester fiber suture (Johnson & Johnson Ethicon Inc, Somerville, NJ, USA). It is available as a regular suture of various calibers, as well as a 5-mm tape with double-ended large blunt needles (**Fig. 1**).[1] It was

Disclaimer: Authors have no financial interests to disclose.
[a] Pennsylvania Hand Center, Bryn Mawr, PA, USA; [b] Orthopaedic and Hand Surgery, Jefferson Medical College, Philadelphia, PA, USA; [c] Hand Therapy Department, Pennsylvania Hand Center, Bryn Mawr, PA, USA
* Corresponding author. Pennsylvania Hand Center, 101 South Bryn Mawr Avenue, Suite 300, Bryn Mawr, PA 19010.
E-mail address: Marwan.Wehbe@pahandcenter.com

hand.theclinics.com

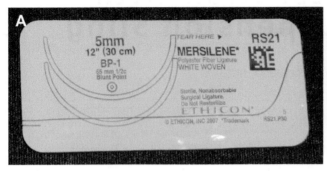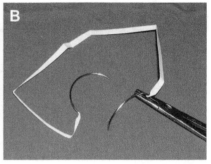

Fig. 1. (A) Packaging of 5-mm wide Mersilene tape. (B) Suture is "double-ended" with blunt semicircular needles and a 12 inch long weaved polyester ribbon. (Courtesy of Pennsylvania Hand Center, Bryn Mawr, PA, USA; with permission.)

initially used to purse-string the incompetent cervix in high-risk pregnancies but has also been used to strengthen repairs in shoulder, open chest surgery, and other locations.[2–4] The in-vitro properties of Mersilene sutures are described in another chapter of this book (A Carpal Ligament Substitute, Part 1, by Martin and Wehbe).

The goal of this procedure is to suspend the base of the first metacarpal to the base of the second metacarpal (Fig. 2). The stability of the second metacarpal will prevent proximal migration of the first metacarpal. The intermetacarpal joint of the second-third metacarpals will prevent the suture from moving proximally. The size and curve of this particular suture make it ideal and easy to pass from the dorsal aspect of the hand, around the base of the second metacarpal, into the wound and around the base of the first metacarpal, with minimal dissection (Fig. 3).

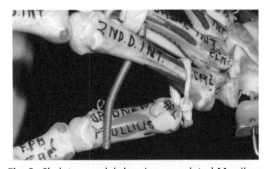

Fig. 2. Skeleton model showing completed Mersilene suspension. The suture passes around the base of the second metacarpal and close to, but not around, the bony part of the first metacarpal. (Courtesy of Pennsylvania Hand Center, Bryn Mawr, PA, USA; with permission.)

SURGICAL TECHNIQUE

A zigzag incision is performed in the dorsoradial aspect of the wrist, to blend the eventual scar with the wrist creases. Dissection is carried through subcutaneous tissues, with great care taken to preserve neurovascular structures. The first dorsal extensor compartment is opened only if there are preoperative signs of De Quervain's disease. The procedure continues between the abductor pollicis longus (APL) and extensor pollicis brevis (EPB). The dorsal branch of the radial artery is identified in that area; it is mobilized and retracted with vessel loops out of harm's way. Trapezial and scaphoid branches are cauterized. Capsule and soft tissues over the trapezium are divided sharply with an I-shaped incision: one transverse incision at the base of the first metacarpal and the other over the distal pole of the scaphoid. Effort must be made to keep from shredding the capsule especially dorsally, because the flaps are necessary for the reconstruction. The trapezium is resected entirely with osteotome and rongeur.

Early on, a wafer of palmar bone was preserved, as recommended by Swanson,[5] to maintain continuity of the capsule for the scaphometacarpal joint. In subsequent years, this step was eliminated, as it was felt that wafer may cause bony impingement in that area, and no ill effects have ensued. Great care must be taken to prevent injury to the flexor carpi radialis (FCR) tendon, which sits inconveniently in a palmar groove of the trapezium, in the depth of the wound. If the FCR tendon is injured during the dissection, it should be repaired because its rupture can result in wrist pain for many weeks. If more than 50% of the tendon is injured, it may be best divided and allowed to retract proximally, to avoid rupture during the

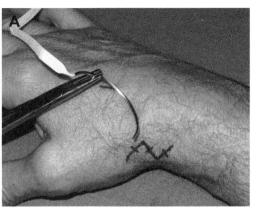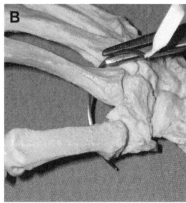

Fig. 3. (A) The Mersilene suture is introduced from a separate dorsal incision and retrieved in the trapezial space. (B) Passage of the Mersilene suture around the base of the second metacarpal is shown on a skeletal model. (*Courtesy of* Pennsylvania Hand Center, Bryn Mawr, PA, USA; with permission.)

postoperative period, which can be alarming to all involved in the rehabilitation phase. Another area of particular attention is the large spur that often projects from the trapezium into the intermetacarpal space and needs to be resected to prevent impingement in that area.

The trapezoid is often ignored in thumb CMC surgery. Degenerative changes between trapezoid and scaphoid are a common cause of failure of surgery for basilar arthritis. That joint needs to be inspected, specifically, or better yet decompressed, and this is accomplished with a partial trapezoidectomy, which is done routinely during this procedure. The portion of the trapezoid that articulates with the scaphoid is resected with an osteotome. Care is taken not to injure the capitate, which is in close proximity. The wrist is taken through its range of motion (ROM) while applying axial loading to it to make sure the remaining portion of the trapezoid does not impinge on the scaphoid in any degree of wrist motion.

A second 1-cm long incision is now performed at the base of the second metacarpal. Minimal blunt dissection is needed to identify the second dorsal interosseous muscle. The Mersilene suture is passed around the base of the second metacarpal and advanced along the palmar aspect of the second and first metacarpals. The tip of the needle is retrieved on the radial side of the first metacarpal base (**Fig. 4**). If the needle cannot be passed in one throw, around the thenar muscle origin, this can be done in 2 steps (**Fig. 5**A, B). A cadaver dissection of the procedure shows that the Mersilene suture actually passes deep to all the muscles and tendons in the palmar aspect of the thumb and index fingers (**Fig. 6**).

The suture is passed through the soft tissues, right against the base of the first metacarpal, and just palmar to the APL insertion. A small portion of the thenar muscle tendinous origin is trapped by the suture as it is passed into the trapezial space, and a few palmar fibers of the APL tendon insertion may also be included within the suture (see **Fig. 5**B). Next, the dorsal part of the suture is passed supraperiosteally from the dorsal wound into the CMC space (**Figs. 7** and **8**). Care is taken to pass the suture deep to the wrist extensor tendons and deep to the radial artery that was previously mobilized. That side of the suture approaches the CMC space over the dorsum of the trapezoid. A square knot is used to tie the suture, which is then cut with a cautery (**Fig. 9**).

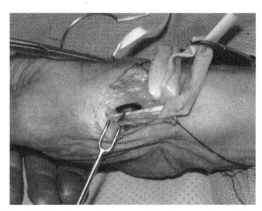

Fig. 4. The size of the needle in question allows passing of the suture around the base of the second and first metacarpals in one throw. (*Courtesy of* Pennsylvania Hand Center, Bryn Mawr, PA, USA; with permission.)

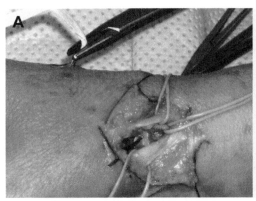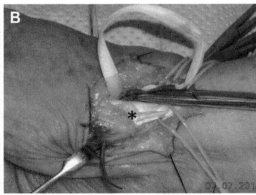

Fig. 5. The palmar part of the suture may be passed in 2 throws if necessary. (*A*) Needle is retrieved in trapezial space. (*B*) Needle is then passed around the base of the first metacarpal through the tendinous origin of the thenar muscles. The suture is passed through the soft tissues, right against the base of the first metacarpal, and just palmar to the APL insertion. (*Asterisk*) shows point of needle re-entry into the trapezial space. (*Courtesy of* Pennsylvania Hand Center, Bryn Mawr, PA, USA; with permission.)

The cautery solders the ends of the suture and prevents unraveling of the polyester weave. The knot and suture ends are now sewn with 2–0 Mersilene sutures to prevent untying.

The knot is tied while an assistant applies some traction to the thumb. The resulting knot ends up inside of the trapezial space. Now axial compression will reveal the adequacy of the suspension (**Fig. 10**). If the suspension is felt to be insufficient, a few more 2–0 Mersilene sutures may be used to further tighten the Mersilene band or to anchor it to the distal part of the FCR tendon, which is in the depth of the wound. Next, the dorsal capsule radial and ulnar flaps are reefed and sutured with 2–0 Mersilene. A tight capsular repair is desirable;

a purse-string type repair that invaginates soft tissue into the trapezial space can provide some soft tissue interposition and possibly help prevent subsidence further.

Radiographs may be obtained intraoperatively and are helpful in early stages of the learning curve for this procedure (**Fig. 11**). They should be obtained before capsule closure to allow any necessary adjustments to the sling before suturing the capsule. A bulky dressing is applied with a thumb spica plaster splint for edema and pain control. Within one week, the patient undergoes dressing change and starts hand therapy. A protective spica splint is used full time except for ROM and hygiene for approximately 6 weeks. Theoretically,

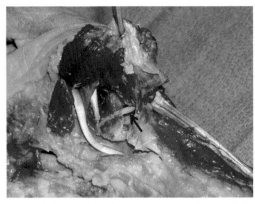

Fig. 6. Cadaver dissection showing position of the Mersilene suture (*arrow*) in the palmar aspect of the hand, deep to all thenar muscles and tendons. (*Courtesy of* Pennsylvania Hand Center, Bryn Mawr, PA, USA; with permission.)

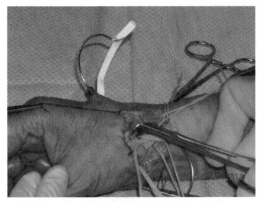

Fig. 7. The dorsal part of the suture is passed into the trapezial space with the help of a Kelly clamp, right on bone, deep to all soft tissue structures. (*Courtesy of* Pennsylvania Hand Center, Bryn Mawr, PA, USA; with permission.)

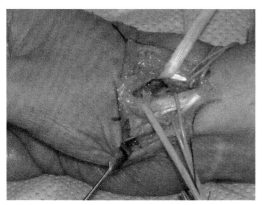

Fig. 8. Both ends of the Mersilene tape are now in the trapezial space. The palmar end is superficial to the capsule, and the dorsal end is deep to the capsular flap. (*Courtesy of* Pennsylvania Hand Center, Bryn Mawr, PA, USA; with permission.)

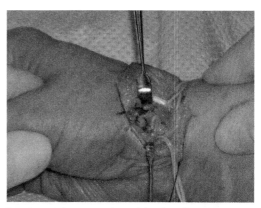

Fig. 10. Axial compression of the thumb at the completion of the procedure demonstrates the strength of the suspension arthroplasty against subsidence. (*Courtesy of* Pennsylvania Hand Center, Bryn Mawr, PA, USA; with permission.)

this is to allow fibrous ingrowth into the polyester sutures, which would serve to permanently reinforce these sutures.

RESULTS

Mersilene suspension sling arthroplasty has been used in 90 hands since 1987. Thirty-eight patients were available for review, with a minimum of 24-months follow-up (range 2–23 years, average 6.78 years). There were 3 men (8%) and 35 women (92%), ages ranging from 37 to 86 years (average 64 years). Thirty-five (92%) were right-handed, and surgery was for the dominant hand in 17 cases (45%) and for both hands in 5 patients (13%).

Preoperative pain ratings ranged between 4 and 6 (on a 10 scale) and became zero at last follow-up in all but 2 patients who rated their pain as 1/10.

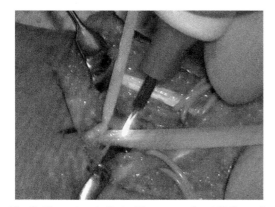

Fig. 9. The suture is tied with a square knot (2 throws), and excess material is cut off with cautery. The knot is then sutured to prevent loosening. (*Courtesy of* Pennsylvania Hand Center, Bryn Mawr, PA, USA; with permission.)

Grip strength improved significantly, and pinch strength increased moderately (**Table 1**). Within one week after surgery, radiographs revealed a scaphoid-first metacarpal distance of 4 to 14 mm (average 8.2 mm). At final follow-up, the average loss of height (subsidence) was 2 mm (range 0–6 mm) (**Table 2**).

These patients had an above average activity level (rated 3.3 out of 5, with 0 being sedentary, and 5 heavy labor). All patients were pleased with their surgery, and 13% of patients returned for surgery on their other hand (**Fig. 12**).

The data were also analyzed to include patients with only 1 year of follow-up. This brought the total to 55 patients with an average follow-up of 5 years (range 1–23 years). All patient demographics, preoperative data and results at final follow-up, were essentially identical except for grip that differed slightly from the cohort with more than two-year follow-up (pre-op grip averaged 35lbs and at final follow-up 47lbs, compared with grips in **Table 1**).

DISCUSSION

Patients with hand arthritis present with degenerative changes in their distal interphalangeal joints, at the thumb base, or both. The importance of thumb use to hand function makes basilar arthritis debilitating. Witness to that is the plethora of techniques that have been developed to deal with that problem. Bone resections and osteotomies, interposition of silicone rubber, polyethylene, pyrocarbon, metal and other spacers, and numerous joint replacements have all had variable results. Another way to look at this problem is that, perhaps, none of these techniques worked well enough or withstood

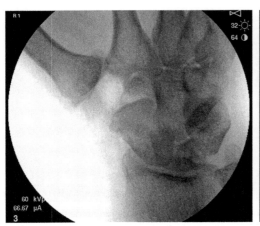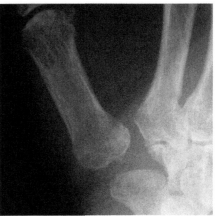

Fig. 11. Intraoperative radiographs demonstrating the complete trapeziectomy and partial trapezoidectomy in 2 different cases. (*Courtesy of* Pennsylvania Hand Center, Bryn Mawr, PA, USA; with permission.)

the test of time to stop the flow of solutions that are still being offered.

Comparing various techniques is difficult for many reasons. Pain and activity level are difficult to gauge and are not necessarily comparable from one study to another, because of patient variables such as personality, activity level in hobbies and work, compliance with treatment, and changes in all these factors over time, especially in an older population. Surgeon variables also affect the outcome with patient selection, change in the details of a procedure over time, and create difficulties in standardization of function and outcome measurements. There is not even an agreement on how to measure thumb ROM!

Many surgeons are performing procedures for thumb CMC arthrosis without much conviction of the importance of that procedure.[6] Furthermore, most studies have a short follow-up (average 12 months) and do not demonstrate any advantage of one procedure over others.[7,8]

Simple excision of the trapezium was described by Gervis in 1949.[9] Although complications surfaced following these early attempts at trapezium resection, Swanson introduced silicone interposition arthroplasty in 1968.[10,11] After initial widespread excitement about that procedure, it fell in disfavor because of implant instability, fragmentation, and silicone synovitis.[12,13] Next came an era of tendon ligament reconstructions using tendon grafts, popularized by Eaton and Littler,[14] as well as Burton and Pellegrini[15] and Weilby.[16] Many variations of that procedure have been reported, with or without a bone tunnel, with or without tendon ("anchovy") interposition, and all seem to yield similar results.[17,18]

Interpositions other than tendons have been attempted with variable success. Available materials were recently reviewed by Birman and Strauch.[19] Artelon, a biodegradable polyurethane urea implant (Artimplant AB, Gothenburg, Sweden), was offered as the ideal interposition material. Its success was

Table 1 Data of 38 Mersilene sling suspension arthroplasties		
	Pre-op	Post-op
Pain (10 scale)	4–6	0–1
Grip (lbs)	0–95 (37)	5–110 (45)
Key Pinch (lbs)	0–23 (9)	2–23 (10)
Pulp Pinch (lbs)	0–16 (7)	2–16 (9)

Averages in parentheses.

Table 2 Radiographic appearance after Mersilene sling suspension arthroplasties	
Scaphometacarpal distance 1 wk post-op	4–14 mm (8.2 mm)
Scaphometacarpal distance at final follow-up	2–10 mm (6 mm)
Height loss (subsidence) at final follow-up	0–6 mm (2 mm)

Averages in parentheses.

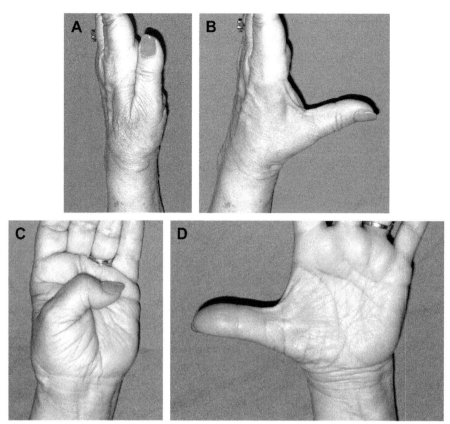

Fig. 12. Patient thumb ROM 10 years after Mersilene sling suspension arthroplasty. (*A*) Neutral position. (*B*) CMC abduction. (*C*) CMC flexion. (*D*) CMC extension. (*Courtesy of* Pennsylvania Hand Center, Bryn Mawr, PA, USA; with permission.)

very short-lived because of mechanical failure and foreign body reactions.[20–22] Other materials were also tried such as acellular dermal allograft (Graft-Jacket; Wright Medical Technology, Inc. Arlington, TN, USA). Early results were, again, similar to other procedures.[23]

Interesting new techniques have been introduced to deal with this vexing problem. Arthroscopic resection of both the CMC and STT joints, with no other intervention, seemed to provide pain relief at one year of follow-up, a very short follow-up for degenerative disease.[24] Although most described procedures use FCR tendon for the suspension, a portion of the APL tendon has been used for suspension,[25] as was the abductor pollicis brevis and opponens pollicis.[26] The extensor carpi radialis longus was also offered as an option followed by casting for 6 weeks.[27] Comprehensive reviews of available techniques seem to always conclude that no technique is superior to others and most have some successes and drawbacks.[28,29]

Beyond spacers, K-wires and other devices have been used to maintain the scaphometacarpal space,[30] sometimes with disastrous results

(tightrope suspension[31]). Most procedures involve postoperative immobilization of 3 to 8 weeks. Although casting up to 6 weeks after trapeziectomy is recommended by some,[27] others have resorted to K-wire fixation for 8 weeks.[32] Surgical time for tendon suspension/interposition is more than 2 hours on average,[33] whereas Mersilene suspension could be done in little more than 1 hour.

Thumb metacarpophalangeal (MP) joint problems must be addressed in a standard fashion as well. Any MP hyperextension deformity should be corrected because zigzag principles dictate that MP hyperextension would force the CMC joint into a flexion posture. It was suggested that hyperextension should be addressed only if it goes beyond 35 degrees,[34] with transection of the EPB to weaken thumb MP extension (with proximal transfer of the EPB to the base of the first metacarpal, to improve thumb CMC abduction), a palmar capsulodesis, or fusion of the MP joint.

The STT joint also requires special consideration. If ignored, it may be a source of continued pain and failed CMC resection arthroplasty.

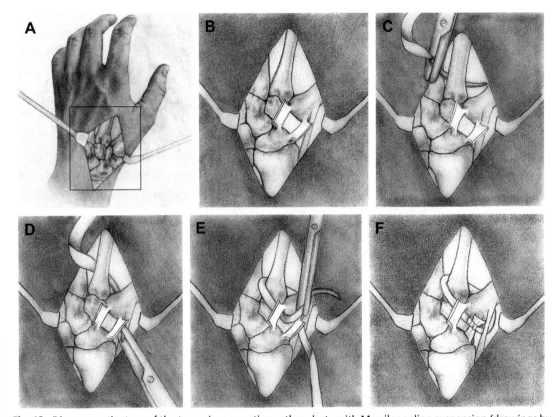

Fig. 13. Diagrammatic steps of the trapezium resection arthroplasty with Mersilene sling suspension (drawings by Marie-Lyne Grenier). (*A*) Surgical approach is through 2 separate incisions, unlike this representation. (*B*) Trapezium resection and partial trapeziectomy completed, with capsule flaps preserved. (*C*) Needle introduced around base of second metacarpal. (*D*) Needle is retrieved over tendinous origin of thenar muscles and deep to APL tendon. (*E*) Dorsal needle is passed deep to all soft tissue structures and retrieved in trapezial space. (*F*) Mersilene tape suture is tied within the trapezial space, trapping the radial half of the dorsal capsule as a purse-string. A palmar slip of the APL tendon may be trapped in the suture, to supplement possible deficiency in that capsule. (*Courtesy of* Pennsylvania Hand Center, Bryn Mawr, PA, USA; with permission.)

STT fusion and trapezoid resection have been described for the treatment of isolated STT arthritis.[35] At the time of trapezium resection, complete trapezoidectomy does not seem to alter wrist biomechanics significantly.[36]

SUMMARY

Trapezium resection arthroplasty with Mersilene sling suspension is a simple and reproducible procedure (**Fig. 13**). It does not require the use of any implants or expensive materials, and it can be easily learned and completed within 90 minutes of tourniquet time. This procedure also does away with prolonged postoperative immobilization and allows the patient to return to normal activity sooner, with improved pain-free ROM and strength. Patients observed up to 23 years have maintained their ROM and strength and are uniformly happy with their outcomes. Our results

also suggest that these patients' condition essentially plateaued by 12 months after surgery.

REFERENCES

1. Available at: http://www.ecatalog.ethicon.com/sutures-non-absorbable/view/mersilene-suture. Accessed October 1, 2012.
2. Tacchi D, Snaith L. The surgical treatment of recurrent late abortion. BJOG 1962;69(4):608–13.
3. Puc MM, Charles H, Antinori CH, et al. Ten-year experience with Mersilene-reinforced sternal wound closure. Ann Thorac Surg 2000;70:97–9.
4. Yang SW, Lin LC, Chang SJ, et al. Treatment of acute unstable distal clavicle fractures with single coracoclavicular suture fixation. Orthopedics 2011;34(6):172–6.
5. Swanson A. Reconstructive surgery in. the arthritic hand and foot. Ciba Clin Symp 1979;31(6):10.
6. Brunton LM, Wilgis EF. A survey to determine current practice patterns in the surgical treatment of advanced

thumb carpometacarpal osteoarthrosis. Hand 2010;5: 415–22.

7. Vermeulen GM, Slijper H, Feitx R, et al. Surgical management of primary thumb carpometacarpal osteoarthritis: a systematic review. J Hand Surg Am 2011;36:157–69.

8. Shuler MS, Luria S, Trumble TE. Basal joint arthritis of the thumb. J Am Acad Orthop Surg 2008;16(7):418–23.

9. Gervis WH. Excision of the trapezium fo osteoarthritis of the trapezio-metacarpal joint. J Bone Joint Surg Br 1949;31:537–739.

10. Conolly WB, Rath S. Revision procedures for complications of surgery for osteoarthritis of the carpometacarpal joint of the thumb. J Hand Surg Br 1993;18:533–9.

11. Swanson AB. Silicone rubber implants for replacement of arthritis or destroyed joints in the hand. Surg Clin North Am 1968;48:1113–27.

12. van Cappelle HG, Deutman R, van Horn JR. Use of the Swanson silicone trapezium implant for treatment of primary osteoarthritis. J Bone Joint Surg Am 2001;83:999–1004.

13. Murray PM, Wood MB. The results of treatment of synovitis of the wrist induced by particles of silicone debris. J Bone Joint Surg Am 1998;80:397–406.

14. Eaton RG, Littler JW. Ligament reconstruction or the painful thumb carpometacarpal joint. J Bone Joint Surg Am 1984;55:1655–66.

15. Burton RI, Pellegrini VD Jr. Surgical management of basal joint arthritis of the thumb: part II. Ligament reconstruction with tendon interposition arthroplasty. J Hand Surg Am 1986;11:324–32.

16. Weilby A. Tendon interposition arthroplasty of the first carpo-metacarpal joint. J Hand Surg Br 1988;13:421–5.

17. Kriegs-Au G, Petje G, Fojtl E, et al. Ligament reconstruction with or without tendon interposition to treat primary thumb carpometacarpal osteoarthritis. J Bone Joint Surg Am 2004;86:209–18.

18. Vermeulen GM, Brink SM, Sluiter J, et al. Ligament reconstruction arthroplasty for primary thumb carpometacarpal osteoarthritis (Weilby technique): prospective cohort study. J Hand Surg Am 2009;34:1393–401.

19. Birman MV, Strauch R. Update on nonautogenous interposition arthroplasty for thumb basilar joint arthritis. J Hand Surg Am 2011;36:2056–9.

20. Joerheim M, Isaxon I, Flondell, et al. Short-term outcomes of trapeziometacarpal Artelon Implant compared with tendon suspension interposition arthroplasty for osteoarthritis: a matched cohort study. J Hand Surg Am 2009;34:1381–7.

21. Giuffrida AY, Gyuricza C, Perino G, et al. Foreign body reaction to Artelon spacer: case report. J Hand Surg Am 2009;34:1388–92.

22. Robinson PM, Muir LT. Foreign body reaction associated with Artelon: report of three cases. J Hand Surg Am 2011;36:116–20.

23. Kokkalis ZT, Zanaros G, Weiser RW, et al. Trapezium resection with suspension and interposition arthroplasty using acellular dermal allograft using acellular dermal allograft for thumb carpometacarpal arthritis. J Hand Surg Am 2009;34:1029–36.

24. Cobb T, Sterbank P, Lemke J. Arthroscopic resection arthroplasty for treatment of combined carpometacarpal and scaphotrapeziotrapezoid (pantrapezial) arthritis. J Hand Surg Am 2011;36:413–9.

25. Sammer DM, Amadio PC. Description of a new technique for thumb basal arthroplasty. J Hand Surg Am 2010;35:1198–205.

26. Heyworth BE, Jobin C, Monica JT, et al. Long-term follow-up of basal joint resection arthroplasty of the thumb with transfer of the abductor pollicis brevis origin to the flexor carpi radialis tendon. J Hand Surg Am 2009;34:1021–8.

27. Illarramendi AA, Boretto JG, Gallucci GL, et al. Trapeziectomy and intermetacarpal ligament reconstruction with the extensor carpi radialis longus for osteoarthritis of the trapeziometacarpal joint: surgical technique and long-term results. J Hand Surg Am 2006;31:1315–21.

28. Kapoutsis DV, Dardas A, Day CS. Carpometacarpal and scaphotrapeziotrapezoid arthritis: arthroscopy, arthroplasty and arthrodesis. J Hand Surg Am 2011;36:354–66.

29. Gangopadhyay S, McKenna H, Burke FD, et al. Five to 18-year follow-up for treatment of trapeziometacarpal osteoarthritis: a prospective comparison of excision, tendon interposition, and ligament reconstruction and tendon interposition. J Hand Surg Am 2012;37:411–7.

30. Yao J, Zlotolow DA, Murdock R, et al. Suture button compared with k-wire fixation for maintenance of posttrapeziectomy space height in a cadaver model of lateral pinch. J Hand Surg Am 2010;35:2061–5.

31. Khalid M, Jones ML. Index metacarpal fracture after tightrope suspension following trapeziectomy: case report. J Hand Surg Am 2012;37:418–22.

32. Kochevar AJ, Adham CN, Adham MN, et al. Thumb basal joint arthroplasty using abductor pollicis longus tendon: an average 5.5-year follow-up. J Hand Surg Am 2011;36:1326–32.

33. Sandwall BJ, Cameron TE, Netsher DT, et al. Basal joint osteoarthritis of the thumb: ligament reconstruction and interposition versus hematoma distraction arthroplasty. J Hand Surg Am 2010;35:1968–75.

34. Poulter RJ, Davis TR. Management of hyperextension of the metacarpo-phalangeal joint in association with trapeziometacarpal joint osteoarthritis. J Hand Surg Br 2011;36:280–4.

35. Garcia-Elias M. Excisional arthroplasty for scaphotrapezialtrapezoidal osteoarthritis. J Hand Surg Am 2011;36:516–20.

36. Wright TW, Thompson J, Conrad BP. Loading of the index metacarpal after trapezial and partial versus complete trapezoid resection. J Hand Surg Am 2006;1:58–62.

Trapezium Prosthetic Arthroplasty (Silicone, Artelon, Metal, and Pyrocarbon)

Mark A. Vitale, MD, MPH[a], Fraser Taylor, MB, BS, FRACS[b,c],
Mark Ross, MB, BS, FRACS[b,c,d], Steven L. Moran, MD[e,*]

KEYWORDS

• Thumb • Trapezial-metacarpal (TM) joint • Silicone • Artelon • Pyrocarbon • Total joint arthroplasty

KEY POINTS

• Trapezium prosthetic arthroplasty has been used to treat basal joint arthritis for nearly 5 decades.
• Implant arthroplasty seeks to preserve joint biomechanics, avoid metacarpal subsidence, and provide immediate stability.
• There has been rapid development of trapezial prosthetic implants, including synthetic interposition materials, metal total joint arthroplasties and pyrocarbon trapezial arthroplasties.
• While many recently available implants have been shown to have short-term success, determining the medium- to long-term outcomes require further study.

INTRODUCTION

The basal joint of the thumb is the second most commonly affected joint by arthritis.[1] Degenerative disease of this joint can result in significant pain, stiffness, weakness, and disability. Conservative measures, such as nonsteroidal anti-inflammatory drugs, splinting, and intra-articular corticosteroid injections, can provide relief for some patients; for those with severe disease in whom nonoperative measures fail, many surgical methods are available, with successful outcomes reported in the literature. These procedures include trapeziectomy alone,[2–4] trapeziectomy and ligament reconstruction with or without tendon interposition,[2,5–9] arthrodesis,[4,10] arthroscopic resection,[11–15] metacarpal extension osteotomy,[16–19] and a variety of methods of prosthetic implant arthroplasty. To date, no single method has emerged superior, although each method has specific advantages and disadvantages for the surgeon to consider.

In contrast to ablative resection and joint fusion procedures, which sacrifice function of the basal joint in an effort to provide pain relief, prosthetic arthroplasty offers the theoretic advantages of preservation of normal anatomy and biomechanics. This could be accomplished without subsidence of the thumb metacarpal, with preservation of normal motion at the trapezialmetacarpal (TM) joint, prevention of metacarpophalangeal joint hyperextension, and immediate stability. Although the results of different joint replacement procedures of the TM joint have been variable with regards to these goals, this review summarizes the history of implant arthroplasty, evolution of prosthetic designs, and outcomes of implants available for use.

This work did not receive any financial support. MR and SLM consult for Integra Life Sciences.
[a] Department of Orthopaedic Surgery, Mayo Clinic, 200 First Street, Rochester, MN 55905, USA; [b] Department of Orthopaedic Surgery, Princess Alexandra Hospital, 199 Ipswich Road, Woolloonabba, Queensland 4102, Australia; [c] Brisbane Hand & Upper Limb Clinic, 9/259 Wickham Terrace, Brisbane, Queensland, 4000, Australia; [d] School of Medicine (Orthopaedic Surgery), The University of Queensland, St Lucia, Queensland, 4067, Australia; [e] Division of Plastic Surgery, Mayo Clinic, 200 First Street, Rochester, MN 55905, USA
* Corresponding author.
E-mail address: moran.steven@mayo.edu

Hand Clin 29 (2013) 37–55
http://dx.doi.org/10.1016/j.hcl.2012.08.020
0749-0712/13/$ – see front matter © 2013 Elsevier Inc. All rights reserved.

Overview/Classification of Trapeziometacarpal Implant Arthroplasty

There is a bewildering array of implants currently available for use in thumb TM implant arthroplasty. The authors propose the following classification scheme in an attempt to bring some order into the assessment and understanding of available options.

Total Replacement

Separate trapezial and metacarpal components

- de la Caffinière (Benoist Girard et Cye, Baguaux, France)
- Braun-Cutter prosthesis (Small Bone Innovations/Avanta Orthopaedics, San Diego, California)
- Avanta Surface Replacement (SR) TM prosthesis (Avanta Orthopaedics)

Hemiarthroplasty

Anatomic

- PyroCarbon Saddle (Integra Life Sciences, Plansboro, NJ)

Nonanatomic

- CMI Carpometacarpal Implant (BioProfile/Tornier, Edina, Minnesota)
- NuGrip (Integra Life Sciences, Plansboro, NJ)
- PyroHemiSphere (Integra Life Sciences, Plansboro, NJ)

Interposition

Partial trapezial resection

- Unconstrained
  ○ PyroSphere (Integra Life Sciences, Plansboro, NJ)
  ○ Pyrocardan (BioProfile/Tornier)
- Constrained
  ○ Artelon (Small Bone Innovations, Morrisville, Pennsylvania)
  ○ PyroDisk (Integra Life Sciences, Plansboro, NJ)

Total trapezial replacement

- Silicone (eg, Swanson [Wright Medical Technology, Arlington, Tennessee])
- Metallic (eg, TrapEZX [Extremity Medical, Parsippany, New Jersey])
- Pyrocarbon
  ○ Pi2 (BioProfile/Tornier)

○ Modified PyroDisk (Integra Life Sciences, Plansboro, NJ)

Silicone

The history of trapezial implant arthroplasty began in the 1960s, when Swanson and colleageus[20] proposed trapeziectomy and silicone arthroplasty to replace a degenerative TM joint. Silicone arthroplasty of the trapezium has been extensively studied over the past 5 decades, and silicone elastomer implants, such as the Swanson endoprosthesis (Wright Medical Technology) have the longest track record of any of the implant arthroplasties for the basal joint (**Fig. 1**).[20] Results have generally been limited by silicone synovitis, secondary instability of the joint, and long-term implant failure.[21–24] On a histologic level, this has been confirmed by the examination of failed silicone implants of the fingers, wrist, and elbow: billions of silicone particles smaller than 15 μm were found in the inflammatory debris surrounding these implants.[25] Furthermore, there have been recent experimental data demonstrating oxidation of silicone elastomer finger metacarpophalangeal and interphalangeal arthroplasty in vivo, which may lead to implant fracture.[26]

The prevalence of silicone synovitis, in the trapezium, specifically, however, has been less common a problem than that reported with carpal and small joint implants in general, although the outcomes have been mixed. In 1986, Pellegrini and Burton published their results of a series of 72 procedures in 53 patients with basal joint osteoarthritis.[6] In a subset of 32 silicone arthroplasties at an average of 3.2-year follow-up, there was

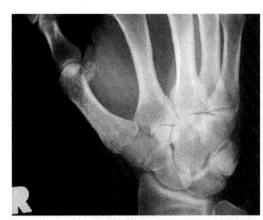

Fig. 1. Posteroanterior radiograph of a TM joint silicone arthroplasty at 5 years postoperatively. (*From* Bezwada HP, Webber JB. Questions regarding the Swanson silicone trapezium implant. J Bone Joint Surg Am 2002;84(5):872; with permission.)

early pain relief but a 50% loss of height and subluxation of the metacarpal, with an average of 35% of the width of the prosthesis. They reported a 25% failure rate and reactive silicone giant cell synovitis with adjacent bone resorption in several cases. The investigators concluded that silicone arthroplasty was not a viable option for osteoarthritis of the basal joint, even though silicone hemiarthroplasty of the trapezium could result in satisfactory outcomes in the low-demand rheumatoid patient. Amadio and colleagues[27] reported on a comparison of a trapezial silicone spacer in 25 patients versus trapeziectomy alone in 25 patients and showed superior results with fewer complications in those with resection arthroplasty at a follow-up, ranging from 1 to 9 years. Lanzetta and Foucher[28] conducted a retrospective study of 85 patients with 98 surgical procedures divided into 3 groups—those receiving Swanson arthroplasties, patients receiving Ashworth-Blatt hemiarthroplasties, and, lastly, patients receiving trapeziectomy with ligament reconstruction and tendon interposition (LRTI). At 5 years, 15% of patients receiving Swanson arthroplasties required surgical revision, and radiographic evidence of silicone synovitis was common with one case requiring surgery secondary to this reaction. Overall, however, the results of both Swanson arthroplasty and LRTI were superior to those of the Ashworth-Blatt hemiarthroplasty.

Lehmann and colleagues[29] compared 27 patients treated with silicone arthroplasty with 75 patients treated with LRTI and found no differences in pain relief, range of motion, or strength between groups, although there was less radiographic subsidence of the thumb metacarpal in the group with silastic interposition. The investigators concluded that given the complication rate reported in other series, silicone arthroplasty should be limited to patients with rheumatoid arthritis in whom maximal preservation of bone stock is desirable. In 1999, Lovell and colleagues[30] retrospectively compared 58 cases of Swanson silicone arthroplasty with 56 cases of LRTI at an average follow-up of 5.2 years. Significantly better results were reported for pain at 1 year as well as patient-reported performance on specific tasks and overall function in those receiving Swanson arthroplasties; patients requiring further surgery or removal of the implant (8 in each group) were, however, excluded from the analysis, a major methodologic flaw, which excluded the worst results from the analysis.

Contemporary series with more rigorous outcome assessments have generally found comparable or poorer results with silicone arthroplasty compared with alternative surgical treatments. In 2002, Tagil and Kopylov[31] reported a prospective, randomized trial of Swanson versus trapeziectomy and abductor pollicis longus (APL) suspension arthroplasty in 26 patients with osteoarthritis of the TM joint with an average follow-up of 3.6 years. There was no incidence of clinically evident silicone synovitis, but bone cysts developed in the metacarpal and the scaphoid and 2 silicone prostheses dislocated early. All 13 patients in the silicone group and 11 of 13 in the APL arthroplasty group reported that they were satisfied, and pain relief was equivalent in both groups, although half of the patients in each group had pain with heavy but not light work. Five of 13 patients in the silicone arthroplasty group had subluxation during stressed pinch. In the same year, Bezwada and Webber[32] reported on the long-term results of 90 silicone arthroplasties of the TM joint in 85 patients at an average of 16.4 years of follow-up. Of the 58 patients available for follow-up (62 implants), 84% of thumbs had satisfactory results with good to excellent pain relief and function. Grip, key pinch, and tip pinch strengths increased on average. Nineteen percent of cases, however, had radiographic subluxation, and implant fracture occurred in 6% requiring revision. The investigators reported that no patients had frank silicone synovitis. In 2003, MacDermid and colleagues[22] reported a series of 26 patients after silicone arthroplasty in which 88% had improvement in pain but with a 20% incidence of revision surgery and 90% rate of radiographic periprosthetic lytic changes at 6.5 years.

In 2005, Minami and colleagues[33] described unsatisfactory long-term results in 12 patients treated with silicone arthroplasty. They reported palmar abduction limited to 23°, with grip strength limited to 9.5 kg, and all but 2 patients had mild to severe pain with a high complication rate, including 2 dislocations and 5 implant failures at an average follow-up period of 15.3 years. Later that year, Taylor and colleagues[11] reported the results of fusion of the TM joint in 36 cases, LRTI in 25 cases, and silastic trapezial replacement in 22 cases. There were no differences in patient satisfaction, pain, range of motion, or tip and key pinch between groups, but there was a higher rate of complications and reoperations in the fusion group.

A cadaveric study of the biomechanical properties of ligament reconstruction with or without tendon interposition compared with a recently developed one-piece silicone elastomer trapezium with fixation into the canal of the metacarpal was reported by Luria and colleagues[34] in 2007 (Tie-In Trapezium Implant, Wright Medical Technology). They showed that the silicone implant had decreased axial and radial displacement and better maintenance of the trapezial space compared with LRTI. This implant did, however, have significant rotation in biomechanical analysis, and no clinical data are yet available.

In addition to trapeziectomy and silicone spacers designed to occupy the entire trapezial space, thin silicone hemiarthroplasty interpositional implants have been available since the 1970s, and these implants have generally been abandoned due to poor results. Ashworth and colleagues[35] studied the use of a modified neurosurgical burr-hole cover as a TM interpositional arthroplasty, but results were poor with some failures due to fracture of the device. Kessler and colleagues[36] later reported on a stemless silicone disc, which was placed between the trapezium and metacarpal and reported several cases with implant dislocation and persistent pain.

Artelon

Artelon (Small Bone Innovations, Morrisville, Pennsylvania) is a T-shaped biodegradable polycaprolactone-based polyurethraneurea material proposed for use in isolated thumb TM arthritis. It was designed to work as both a joint interposition spacer with the vertical spacer portion of the device being placed between the thumb metacarpal base and distal trapezium and as a ligament stabilizer with 2 T-shaped wings of the implant being placed horizontally along the joint to augment the dorsal capsule and prevent dorsoradial migration of the proximal metacarpal (**Fig. 2**). The wings of the implant are typically fixed with 2 2.0-mm cortical screws. In vitro degradation

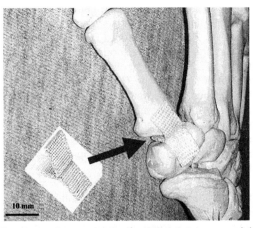

Fig. 2. Artelon spacer in the TM joint in a model. (*From* Nilsson A, Liljensten E, Bergström C, et al. Results from a degradable TM joint Spacer (Artelon) compared with tendon arthroplasty. J Hand Surg Am 2005;30A:380–90; with permission.)

studies have shown that complete hydrolysis of Artelon takes approximately 6 years.[37] Initial reports with this implant showed promise and compared favorably to LRTI. In 2005 Nilsson and colleagues[38] described their initial experience with this implant in 15 patients—10 treated with the Artelon spacer and 5 treated with trapeziectomy and APL stabilization. At 3 years, all patients in both groups were pain-free, and patients treated with the Artelon spacer demonstrated increased key pinch and tripod pinch. A pathologic specimen from one patient at 6 months postoperatively revealed incorporation of the spacer into adjacent bone without signs of foreign body reaction.

The use of Artelon has been described by Badia[16] as a spacer in conjunction with arthroscopic debridement of the trapezium in a level V surgical technique. The investigator purported possible benefits of a minimally invasive technique with potentially less pain and faster recovery as well as trapezial preservation. A 1.9-mm arthroscope is used for visualization, a 2.9-mm burr is used to remove 3 mm of subchondral bone, and then the Artelon spacer is folded and introduced into the TM joint via extension of the portal longitudinally or via insertion through a rigid cannula. The TM joint may be fixed with a Kirschner wire, which the investigator speculated may prevent micromotion and assist in fibrous ingrowth of the implant. No attempt was made to assess patient outcomes or complications.

In more rigorous investigation of patient outcome, longer-term results of Artelon arthroplasty have not been favorable. Jorheim and colleagues[39] reported the results of a matched cohort study of 53 patients comparing 13 patients treated with Artelon arthroplasty versus 40 patients treated with trapeziectomy and LRTI (using APL) in patients with Eaton stages I to III disease. At 13 months, there were no significant differences in the Disabilities of the Arm, Shoulder, and Hand (DASH) questionnaire or pain scores between groups. Those treated with Artelon were 4 times less likely to be satisfied than those treated with LRTI, and 2 patients in the Artelon group were revised to LRTI, with another 2 having revision surgery for screw removal secondary to pain. Additionally, those treated with Artelon had a lower median grip and pinch strength compared with the LRTI group, which the investigators propose would likely have reached significance with a sufficient sample size.

As a follow-up to a pilot study, a randomized, controlled multicenter trial published in 2010 by Nilsson and colleagues[40] studied 109 patients with osteoarthritis of the basal joint treated at 7 different centers in Sweden. Seventy-two patients were treated with the Artelon spacer, and 37 patients were treated with trapeziectomy and LRTI (using either APL, extensor carpi radialis longus, or the Burton procedure). Pain and postoperative swelling were more common in patients treated with Artelon than those treated with LRTI. Additionally, 8% of patients treated with Artelon had subsequent removal of their implants. In contrast to the initial results, there was no increase in key pinch or tripod pinch strength. Although both groups experienced significant improvement in DASH scores and pain relief, those treated with LRTI had significantly better pain relief than those treated with Artelon arthroplasty.

Several case reports have emerged from the literature describing foreign body reactions with use of Artelon in the TM joint, and this reaction may be more common than reported in initial studies. Choung and Tan[41] described a patient with swelling, pain and radiographic osteolysis 10 weeks after an Artelon arthroplasty mimicking infection, with the end result implant removal and multiple surgical synovectomies and a biopsy revealing acute and chronic inflammatory synovitis with multinucleated giant cells. Giuffrida and colleagues[42] similarly reported a patient with painful synovitis and trapezial erosion after implantation of the Artelon spacer into the scaphotrapezial-trapezoidal joint, requiring removal of the implant and revision to LRTI. Biopsy of the soft tissue and synovium revealed a granulomatous foreign body giant cell reaction to the Artelon implant (**Fig. 3**). Additionally, Robinson and

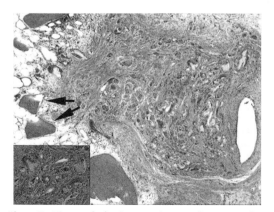

Fig. 3. Histopathologic specimen demonstrating a granulomatous reaction to Artelon with numerous foreign body giant cells in the trapezium bone. Bony trabeculae are shown at left (*arrows*), and the foreign material is shown in the inset under polarized light (hematoxylin-eosin stain, ×200 magnification). (*From* Giuffrida AY, Gyuricza C, Perino G, et al. Foreign body reaction to artelon spacer: case report. J Hand Surg Am 2009;34(8):1388–92; with permission.)

Muir.[43] reported on 3 cases of persistent pain after Artelon TM implant arthroplasty, all requiring removal of the implant and trapeziectomy to resolve symptoms.[43] In all 3 cases, biopsy specimen revealed a foreign-body type reaction with giant cells containing material that was presumed to be Artelon.

Metallic

Numerous metal total joint implant designs have been devised for the treatment of prosthetic replacement of TM arthritis, including various combinations of metal and polyethylene components. The earliest implant was designed by de la Caffinière and Aucouturier, which is a cemented ball-and-socket implant with a polyethylene cup inserted into the trapezium and a cobalt-chromium stem in the metacarpal (Benoist Girard et Cye S.A., Baguaux, France). These investigators reported their early results in 1979, which showed that outcomes were not as good for patients with a primary complaint of stiffness preoperatively but superior outcomes in patients who were indicated for pain and instability.[44] There has been extensive experience with this prosthesis reported in the European literature since this initial study, with overall good clinical results, although there have been several cases of asymptomatic radiographic loosening seen in the trapezial component.[45–50]

Other data, however, brought use of this prosthesis into question because some series have found unacceptably high rates of implant loosening, which did eventually require revision, particularly in younger patients and in men who may put more stress on the prosthesis. van Cappelle and colleagues[48] examined the results of 77 de la Caffinière prostheses implanted for osteoarthritis of the TM joint. At 16 years, the survival rate of the implant was 72%, and the overall loosening rate was 44% (**Fig. 4**). Half of the cases of loosening (more common in men and younger women) were treated with revision, and these patients did significantly poorer. De Smet and colleagues[51] conducted a retrospective survey on 43 de la Caffinière prostheses in 40 patients. Although patients had a 70% satisfaction rate, good range of motion, and increased postoperative grip and pinch force, there was an alarmingly high rate of loosening for this prosthesis (44%). There was a relationship between loosening and younger age. De Smet and colleagues[52] also compared key pinch strength between 26 patients treated with de la Caffinière prosthetic total joint arthroplasty versus 27 patients treated with LRTI with the hypothesis that total joint arthroplasty would

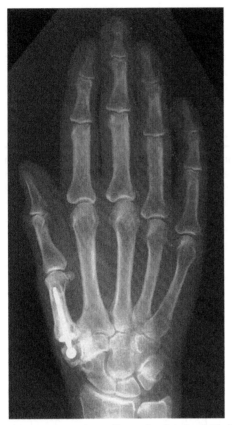

Fig. 4. Posteroanterior radiograph of de la Caffinière prosthesis at 15 years postoperatively revealing loosening of both cup and stem with dislocation. Note the vertical position of the metal ring of the cup, indicating migration and rotation of the cup and dislocation of the components. Despite the radiographic appearance this patient had excellent clinical and subjective scores. (*From* van Cappelle HG, Elzenga P, van Horn JR. Long-term results and loosening analysis of de la Caffinière replacements of the trapeziometacarpal joint. J Hand Surg Am 1999;24(3):476–82; with permission.)

provide better pinch strength; there was, however, no difference between the 2 procedures in key pinch at an average of 2.1 years after surgery, failing to provide support for one of the purported benefits of joint arthroplasty, and there was a 51% loosening rate in this series.

Similar ball-and-socket prosthetic designs were independently devised by Steffee and Nahigian.[53,54] The Steffee prosthesis was a cemented prosthesis with a cobalt-chromium-molybendum alloy metacarpal stem, which articulates with a trapezial ultra–high-molecular-weight polyethylene cup (Laure Prosthetics, Portage, Michigan). Ferrari and Steffee[53] retrospectively reported on the first 45 cases in 38 patients with a follow-up ranging from 2 to 6.5 years. The investigators reported

a 93% rate of pain relief and restoration of range of motion and strength, but 30% of cases had asymptomatic radiolucent lines around the trapezial component (**Fig. 5**). There were 3 cases of symptomatic loosening. In 1999, Hannula and Nahigian[54] described a retrospective report of a different cementless ball-and-socket total joint implant for the TM joint designed with a titanium alloy coated stem and trapezium with a cobalchrome ball articularting with a polyethylene socket (Techmedica, Camarillo, California). The results of this prosthesis were reported in 42 cases in 36 patients with an average 4-year follow-up (**Fig. 6**).[54] They reported 78% good to excellent results. Five cases, however, required revision surgery, and radiolucent lines were also noted in 52% of patients (12 of 13 in the trapezial component), confirming the results by Ferrari and Steffee. Neither of these implants is currently available today.

The GUEPAR (Benoit-Gerrard et Cye S.A., Baguaux, France) prosthesis is a French-designed cemented cobalt-chrome on polyethylene total joint implant with several positive reports in the French and German literature.[55–58] The stem is a smooth monobloc component that is conical in profile and triangular in cross-section with a collar that rests against the metacarpal surface. Masmejean and colleagues[57] showed good clinical midterm results for the second generation of this implant and found that radiolucent lines had no impact on outcome. In 2009, Lemoine and colleagues[59] described the results of the second generation of this prosthesis in 72 patients at a mean follow-up of 4.2 years (**Fig. 7**). There was only a 1.3% revision rate in this series, and 60% of patients were pain-free, with another 18% having pain only with significant activity.

The Elektra prosthesis (Small Bone Innovations, Péronnas, France) is a ball-and-socket semimodular, unconstrained, cementless hydroxyapatite-coated prosthesis (**Fig. 8**). In 2006, Regnard reported on the first 100 patients at an average follow-up of 4.4 years.[60] There were good outcomes documented by improvements in strength, range of motion, and pain relief; 15% of patients, however, had loosening of the cup, and some patients sustained subsidence of the distal component and dislocation. These early results have been attributed to the first generation of implant design and an early technique, which did not involve fixation of the cup or intraoperative fluoroscopy to verify cup orientation. A subsequent prospective study published in 2008 by Ulrich-Vinter and colleagues[61] comparing the Elektra prosthesis with trapeziectomy and APL tendon interposition followed 98 patients at 3, 6,

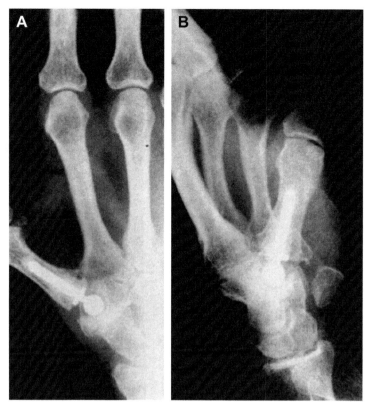

Fig. 5. Posteroanterior (*A*) and lateral (*B*) radiographs of the right thumb of a 73-year-old woman with osteoarthritis 9 years after a Steffee TM prosthesis. (*From* Ferrari B, Steffee AD. Trapeziometacarpal total joint replacement using the Steffee prosthesis. J Bone Joint Surg Am 1986;68(8):1177–84; with permission.)

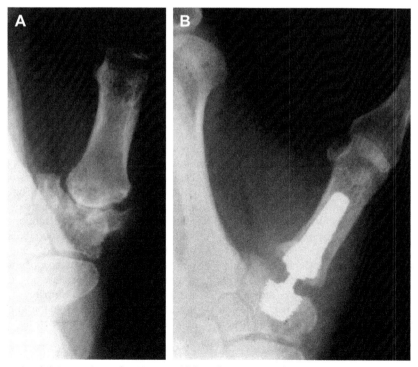

Fig. 6. Preoperative (*A*) Bett's view of a 58-year-old female patient with primary osteoarthritis of the TM joint, and postoperative (*B*) view with a well-positioned titanium total joint prosthetic arthroplasty 25 months postoperatively. (*From* Hannula TT, Nahigian SH. A preliminary report: cementless trapeziometacarpal arthroplasty. J Hand Surg Am 1999;24(1):92–101; with permission.)

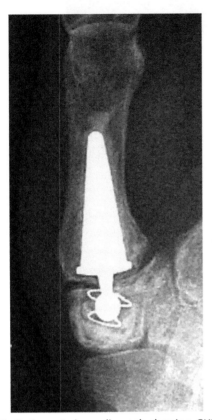

Fig. 7. Posteroanterior radiograph showing GUEPAR prosthesis with complete radiolucent line around trapezial cup in an asymptomatic patient. (*From* Lemoine S, Wavreille G, Alnot JY, et al. Second generation GUEPAR total arthroplasty of the thumb basal joint: 50 months follow-up in 84 cases. Orthop Traumatol Surg Res 2009; 95(1):63–9; with permission.)

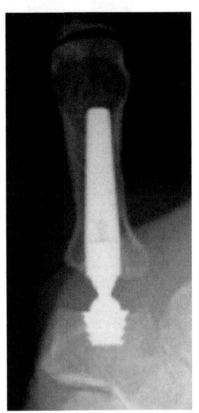

Fig. 8. Elektra total joint prosthesis seen on Posteroanterior radiograph at 1-year follow-up. Osseous integration and fixation of the prosthetic component appear without periprosthetic osteolysis or subluxation of prosthesis. (*From* Ulrich-Vinther M, Puggaard H, Lange B. Prospective 1-year follow-up study comparing joint prosthesis with tendon interposition arthroplasty in treatment of trapeziometacarpal osteoarthritis. J Hand Surg Am 2008;33(8): 1369–77; with permission.)

and 12 months postoperatively and showed excellent results of this prosthesis. The group receiving the total joint arthroplasty had faster and better pain relief, stronger grip strength, improved range of motion, and faster convalescence than the tendon interposition arthroplasty group. At 1 year, osteolysis was evident in the proximity of 2 cups but there were no signs of implant loosening. There was no difference in complications between the 2 groups.

The Braun-Cutter prosthesis (Small Bone Innovations/Avanta Orthopaedics) is a cemented prosthesis with a titanium collarless stem and a polyethylene cup designed for use in Eaton stages III and IV basal joint disease (Fig. 9). Braun reported in 1982 his initial experience in 22 patients with 29 involved TM joints with acceptable results,[62] but there have been significant changes in implant design, cementing techniques and surgical techniques since then, prompting a study by Badia and Sambandam[63] to re-evaluate this

implant. The investigators reported in 2006 on 26 Braun-Cutter TM arthroplasties in a patient cohort with an average of 71 years of age at an average of 3.8 years of follow-up.[63] The results were encouraging, with 96% of patients pain-free at follow-up. Excellent range of motion of 60° of radial abduction and improved pinch (85% of contralateral thumb) were observed. One patient was revised due to posttraumatic loosening, and radiographic analysis at final follow-up did not show any subsequent atraumatic implant loosening. The investigators concluded that this implant is reliable for use in elderly, low-activity patients with advanced TM disease.

The Ledoux prosthesis (Dimso, Marmande, France) is a Belgian design consisting of an uncemented ball-and-socket with the trapezial component having a cylindrical exterior shape and conical interior with a cylindrical polyethylene

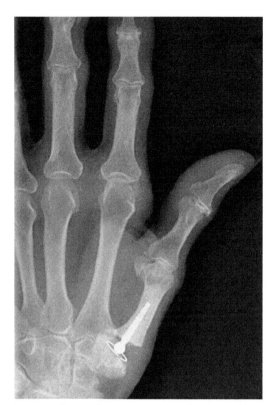

Fig. 9. Well-seated Braun-Cutter total joint prosthesis seen on lateral radiograph at final follow-up without evidence of implant loosening. (*From* Badia A, Sambandam SN. Total joint arthroplasty in the treatment of advanced stages of thumb carpometacarpal joint osteoarthritis. J Hand Surg Am 2006;31(10):1605–14; with permission.)

inlay. The trapezial component is secured both by a screw and boney ingrowth. Although initial reports were encouraging, reports of implant failure prompted a multicenter study by LeDoux[64] where the investigator identified 24 failed prostheses in 188 cases (12.7% failure rate) among 11 surgeons. The investigator sought to determine the cause of failure in these cases. There were 10 cases of improper cup orientation, which caused loosening of the trapezial component. Five cases had subsidence of the stem into the metacarpal medullary canal, and there were 2 cases of stem malalignment. Three cases had a stem that was deemed to be too small. Once case was a septic loosening and 3 dislocations were seen. Twenty-three of the 24 cases were revised, and metallosis of the periprosthetic tissues was seen in 6 of these cases. Ledoux described some modifications to the initial design of the prosthesis to avoid these modes of failure, including treatment of the prosthesis head with ionic nitrogen to prevent metallosis and increasing the range of motion in the

prosthesis to compensate for improper cup orientation. Wachtl and colleagues[49] performed a retrospective review on 88 total metal arthroplasties of the RM joint in 84 patients with either the cemented de la Caffinière prosthesis (43 joints) at a mean follow-up of 63 months versus the revised design cementless Ledoux prosthesis (45 joints) at a mean follow-up of 25 months (**Fig. 10**). Kaplan-Meier analysis revealed that the de la Caffinière prosthesis had a 66.4% survival at 68 months and the Ledoux prosthesis had a 58.9% survival at 16 months, with similarly high rates of both stem and cup components in both designs. The investigators concluded that the currently available contrained ball-and-socket TM prostheses studied at that time were not suitable for use.

Cooney and colleagues[65] developed another TM total joint prosthesis, which was a cemented implant in which the trapezial metal component was a pedestal with a sphere to articulate with a polyethylene-stemmed metacarpal socket (**Fig. 11**); the investigators described this as a surface replacement arthroplasty. This design is a reversed ball-and-socket arrangement, and was developed based on biomechanical studies with 3-D motion analysis using a magnetic Isotrak system comparing the normal TM joint with excision arthroplasty and surface replacement.[66,67] Biomechanical analysis showed that the total joint surface replacement best duplicated thumb

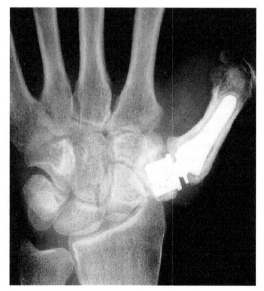

Fig. 10. Posteroanterior radiograph of a Ledoux cementless prosthesis at 3 years postoperatively. (*From* Wachtl SW, Guggenheim PR, Sennwald GR. Cemented and non-cemented replacements of the trapeziometacarpal joint. J Bone Joint Surg Br 1998;80(1):121–5; with permission.)

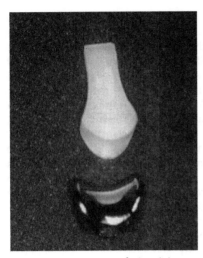

Fig. 11. The Cooney TM resurfacing joint prosthesis represented a saddle joint with biconcave reciprocating articular surfaces and a limited degree of internal joint stability. The trapezial component is made of Co-Cr alloy and the metacarpal stem is made of high-density polyethylene. (*From* Uchiyama S, Cooney WP, Nieber G, et al. Biomechanical analysis of the trapeziometacarpal joint after surface replacement arthroplasty. J Hand Surg Am 1999;24(3):483–90; with permission.)

kinematics whereas trapeziectomy altered the moment arms and center of rotation. Initial clinical data by Cooney and colleagues[65] showed excellent motion and pinch strength but noted that 36% of their implants developed heterotopic bone postoperatively, which had an adverse impact on outcome. They reported that preoperative heterotopic bone, adjacent joint fusion or adjacent joint disease, and poor bone stock all resulted in poor outcomes in their experience, and, as a result, these are contraindications to total joint arthroplasty.

Another surface replacement design is the Avanta SR TM prosthesis (Avanta Orthopaedics), which consists of trapezial and thumb metacarpal base

resurfacing articulations. The trapezial component is made of a cobalt chrome alloy with a peg centered in the trapezium, and the metacarpal component is made of ultra–high-molecular-weight polyethylene (**Fig. 12**). Each component has pegs that are cemented into the medullary canal of its bone. In contrast to the ball-and-socket designs, this implant better replicated the surface anatomy of the normal saddle joint. The first study with this implant by Pérez-Úbeda and colleagues[68] in 20 cases had a high rate of complications at an average of 2.8 years of follow-up, with a 55% rate of loosening and 15% rate of ankylosis secondary to periprosthetic calcifications (**Fig. 13**). Twenty percent of patients needed revision to a salvage procedure, and only 40% of patients had good to excellent results at the end of the study. A recent series by van Rijn and Gosens[69] published in 2010, however, re-evaluated this prosthesis and revealed encouraging results. In 15 cases of prosthetic replacement with the Avanta SR TM implant with an average follow-up of 3 years, the investigators found significantly decreased pain during activitiy and significantly improved function with both hands after surgery as assessed by the sequential occupational dexterity assessment and the Michigan Hand Outcomes Questionnaire. There was no sign of radiographic implant loosening, but there was one implant failure in this series. There was no improvement in range of motion, strength, or function of the operated hand used alone.

In contrast to the metal total joint prosthetic designs, hemiarthroplasty titanium implants have also been used, first devised by Swanson in 1985. In 1997, Swanson and colleagues[70] published the results of 105 Swanson titanium condylar hemiarthroplasty prostheses (Wright Medical Technology) with an average follow-up of 5 years. They reported improvements in motion and strength at 6 months, bone remodeling radiographically, and stability of the implant. There was

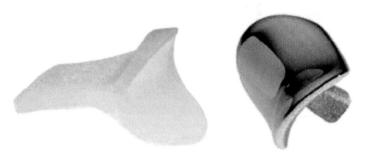

Fig. 12. The Avanta SR TM prosthesis consists of 2 components whose saddle-like articular surfaces have slightly greater curvature than the anatomic surfaces to increase the stability of the articulation. The trapezial component is a Co-Cr alloy with a rounded peg to be seated in the center of the trapezium and the metacarpal component is made of ultra–high-molecular-weight polyethylene. (*From* van Rijn J, Gosens T. A cemented surface replacement prosthesis in the basal thumb joint. J Hand Surg Am 2010;35(4):572; with permission.)

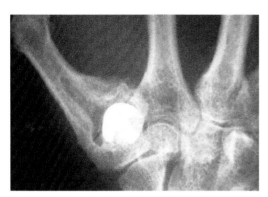

Fig. 13. Posteroanterior radiograph showing an Avanta SR TM replacement in which ankylosis developed after 26 months secondary to periprosthetic calcifications. Despite the radiographic appearance and decreased range of motion, the patient was reported to have complete pain relief. (*From* Pérez-Úbeda MJ, García-López A, Marco Martinez F, et al. Results of the cemented SR trapeziometacarpal prosthesis in the treatment of thumb carpometacarpal osteoarthritis. J Hand Surg Am 2003;28(6):917–25—image originally published by the American Society for Surgery of the Hand; with permission.)

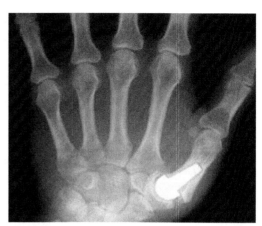

Fig. 14. Posteroanterior radiograph showing titanium TM hemiarthroplasty with typical varus drift of the implant pistoning loose within the metacarpal shaft. (*From* Naidu SH, Kulkarni N, Saunders M. Titanium basal joint arthroplasty: a finite element analysis and clinical study. J Hand Surg Am 2006;31(5):760–5; with permission.)

no sign of wear at 5 years, although other investigators have not been able to reproduce these excellent results. In 2003, Phaltankar and Magnussen reported on 19 titanium hemiarthroplasties in 18 patients at 2.9 years of follow-up, with good pain relief in only 13 cases.[71] Radiographic loosening was seen in 5 cases and trapezial wear was seen in 10 cases, although neither radiographic finding correlated with clinical outcome. One case required revision to trapeziectomy. Naidu and colleagues[72] recently reported on titanium hemiarthroplasty in a 2-part study consisting of a biomechanical finite element analysis and a clinical study in 47 patients with 2 years of follow-up. In the finite element analysis, they showed pistoning behavior with maximum stress concentration in the midmetacarpal shaft and with rotation of the convex sphere of the implant out of the trapezial crater. The clinical analysis had strict inclusion criteria of patients with Eaton stage III arthritis and good bone stock without contractures at the TM or metacarpophalangeal joint. Despite these narrow indications, they showed failure in 10 patients at 9 months, all converted to LRTI. Implant settling occurred mainly in 2 patterns—varus drift and axial subsidence (**Fig. 14**). Titanium is approximately 1000 times stiffer than host bone, and the investigators hypothesized that the modulus mismatch between titanium and host hone was responsible for the high localized stresses seen at the distal tip of the implant. Those without implant failure had

significant improvements in DASH scores, although there was still persistent weakness at 2-year follow-up and the operated thumbs never reached the strength of the contralateral thumbs. All patients who had an LRTI on the contralateral side definitely preferred the side treated with LRTI rather than titanium hemiarthroplasty. The investigators concluded that although titanium arthroplasty may have a role in low-demand patients with sufficient bone stock, high failure rates have prompted them to stop using this prosthesis.

In 2009 a new anatomic metal trapezial replacement called the TrapEZX (Extremity Medical) was designed in conjunction with Amy Ladd, Peter Weiss, and John Faillace. It combines anatomic design with potential for soft tissue ingrowth and suture anchor stabilization (**Fig. 15**). The device has been implanted in more than 100 patients. Although early results have been encouraging (Ladd & Weiss, personal data, 2010-2012), no published data are available for this prosthesis and further evaluation is required.

Pyrolytic Carbon

Pyrolytic carbon is another material that has more recently been developed for use in TM arthroplasty. This is a synthetic material formed by pyrolysis of a hydrocarbon gas. Unlike silicone, Artelon, and titanium, the modulus of elasticity of pyrolytic carbon is similar to that of cortical bone, which theoretically may prevent subsidence and better mimic the native biomechanical properties of the

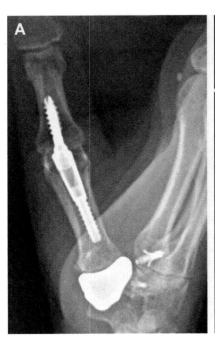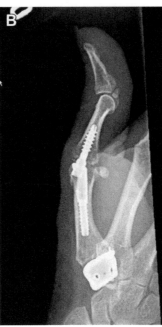

Fig. 15. Posteroanterior (*A*) and lateral radiographs (*B*) of TrapEZX anatomic metallic trapezial total replacement. (Personal image *courtesy of* Mark Ross.)

native TM joint. An additional benefit of pyrolytic carbon may be the potential adherence of certain joint boundary lubrication molecules to its surface, specifically phospholipids, which have been identified as a significant component of synovial fluid lubrication.[73–75] In 1989, Cook and colleagues[76] published a canine hip hemiarthroplasty study, which demonstrated significantly superior acetabular cartilage preservation when articulating against a pyrolytic carbon femoral head compared with a metal femoral head. Early data in primates have revealed no evidence of wear or wear debris or inflammatory synovitis.[77]

Although the use of pyrocarbon has been extensively studied in other small joints of the hand and wrist,[78–87] there are fewer published data describing trapezial arthroplasty. Pyrolytic carbon anatomic interposition arthroplasty has been described by Bellemère and colleagues.[88] The Pyrocardan implant (BioProfile/Tornier) is indicated for Eaton stage I or II disease. The biconcave implant is inserted free into the TM joint with minimal bone resection (**Fig. 16**). Prospective review of a continuous series of 27 implants with follow-up of 12 to 27 months (mean 16.6 months) demonstrated excellent improvements in pain and subjective scores. All implants remained in situ and no complications or revision surgery were reported.[88]

The PyroDisk (Integra Life Sciences) pyrolytic carbon nonanatomic interposition implant is

a biconcave disk with a central hole to allow stabilization with a tendon. Early unpublished results as part of an investigational device trial showed promise. There has been mixed experience with the device in Europe. The PyroDisk has also been implanted as an interposition with complete trapeziectomy. This modified technique has been reported by Stabler.[89] It involves complete trapeziectomy and implantation of the PyroDisk combined with ligament reconstruction and stabilization using the flexor carpi radialis tendon (**Fig. 17**). In a large series of 109 implants, excellent results have been described, although follow-up remains short and further study is required.

A further pyrolytic carbon interposition in association with complete trapeziectomy has also been reported by Ardouin and Bellemère.[90] The Pi2 (BioProfile/Tornier) prosthesis is an oval spacer designed to replace the excised trapezium (**Fig. 18**). Unlike the PyroDisk technique of Stabler, the Pi2 is not stabilized, because the philosophy is to have a free moving adaptive implant. This involves some additional technical requirements in terms of capsuloplasty and/or ligamentoplasty to stabilize the implant. A prospective study of 42 implants in 39 patients demonstrated excellent pain relief and patient satisfaction. Although there were 2 subluxations, none of the implants had been revised at a mean follow-up of 63 months. Another recent

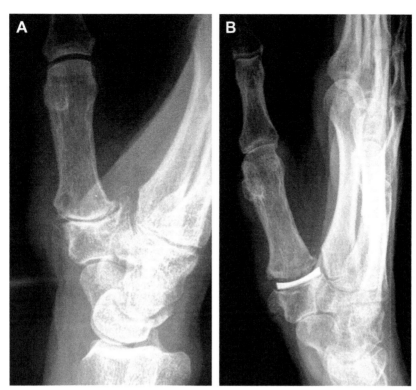

Fig. 16. Preoperative (*A*) and postoperative (*B*) radiograph of Pyrocardan pyrolytic carbon anatomic interposition implant. (*Courtesy of* Philippe Bellemère, Nantes Assitance Main, Clinique Jeanne D'Arc, Nantes, France; with permission.)

study by van Aaken and colleagues[91] reported on 41 patients (45 joints) with at minimum 1-year follow-up. They found that the 73% of patients who were very satisfied with their results and had improved pinch strength and Kapandji scores postoperatively. There was, however, a high failure rate of the prosthesis, with 27% having undergone subsequent removal of the prosthesis at a mean of 11 months postoperatively.

The currently available pyrolytic carbon hemiarthroplasty prosthesis, called the NuGrip (Integra Life Sciences), is a partial trapezial resurfacing implant with a stem that seats in the proximal metacarpal and insets into the trapezium, which is reamed to accept the spherical proximal surface of the implant (**Fig. 19**). The first generation of this prosthesis, which was called the PyroHemi-Sphere, was the proximal component of the pyrocarbon metacarpophalangeal joint implant (originally manufactured by Ascension Orthopedics) used as a TM prosthesis, but the more recently designed implant (NuGrip, Integra Life Sciences) has been designed specifically for TM arthroplasty. In contrast to metal total joint implants with a constrained trapezial component

subjected to high stresses, which may contribute to high loosening rates in clinical series, this implant instead articulates with a hemisphere of subchondral trapezial bone. This obviates the trapezial component loosening, which can lead to revision with total joint prostheses. Ligament stability is crucial to avoid subluxation of the implant, and significant ligamentous instability is a contraindication to use of this implant. This implant is indicated for Eaton stages II and III disease. Scaphotrapezial-trapezoidal joint arthritis is another contraindication to its use. A series from the Mayo Clinic reported in 2009 early outcomes of patients treated with pyrolytic carbon hemiarthroplasty of the TM joint.[92] Fifty-four TM joints in 49 patients were treated, with underlying diagnoses of osteoarthritis in 44 thumbs, rheumatoid arthritis in 8 thumbs, psoriatic arthritis in 1 thumb, and juvenile rheumatoid arthritis in 1 thumb. At 1.8 years, the overall survival rate was 80%. There were 10 patients with metacarpal subluxation, and 7 of these were salvaged by revision surgery to deepen the trapezial cup. Overall there was a high reoperation rate, with 15 reoperations in this series due to dislocation and/or persistent

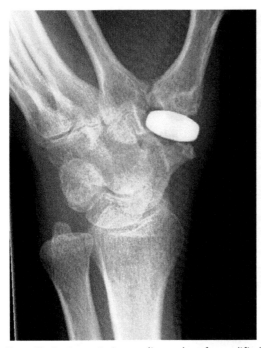

Fig. 17. Posteroanterior radiograph of modified PyroDisk nonanatomic interposition implant with complete trapeziectomy and ligament stabilization. (Personal image *courtesy of* David Stabler, Gold Coast, Queensland, Australia.)

pain. Satisfaction was 81%, and 71% of patients were pain-free whereas 12% reported mild to occasional pain with repetitive activities. Grip strength recovered to 86%, key pinch to 92%, and opposition pinch strength to 95% of the contralateral side. The investigators concluded that, although there was a high complication rate

with subluxation attributed to a shallow trapezial cup in some cases performed early in the learning curve, this may be an acceptable option for treatment of TM arthritis because loosening and subsidence were not seen in this series.

Another recent prospective cohort comparative study of trapeziectomy alone versus trapeziectomy and pyrocarbon hemiarthroplasty by Colegate-Stone and colleagues[93] assessed outcomes in 38 consecutive patients with primary TM joint arthritis. Patients were evaluated with the *Quick-DASH* and a visual analog pain scale, and objective measures included grip strength measurements. They found no significant difference between the 2 groups at 6 or 12 months postoperatively but did find a higher complication rate in the pyrocarbon group, 7 of which sustained complications.

Other Implants

There are several other implants recently been reported in the literature with either limited clinical experience or poor performance limiting widespread use. Use of the ceramic sphere implant called Orthosphere (Wright Medical Technology) manufactured of zirconia ceramic as a spacer between the thumb metacarpal and trapezium was reported by Athwal and colleagues[94] with subsidence in 6 of 7 cases and 1 case with implant dislocation requiring revision to trapeziectomy (**Fig. 20**). This implant was again recently reviewed by Adams and colleagues.[95] In their series of 50 patients, trapezium fracture was evident in 15, erosion of the implant into the trapezium in 11, and other complications in 10 over a 3-year follow-up. Gore-Tex (polytetrafluoroethylene) synthetic interposition arthroplasty (W.L. Gore

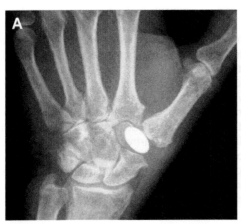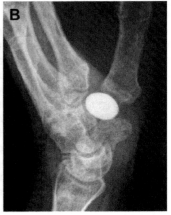

Fig. 18. Posteroanterior (*A*) and lateral (*B*) radiographs of the Pi2 pyrocarbon prosthesis in a patient 3 years postoperatively. (*Courtesy of* Philippe Bellemère, Nantes Assitance Main, Clinique Jeanne D'Arc, Nantes, France; with permission.)

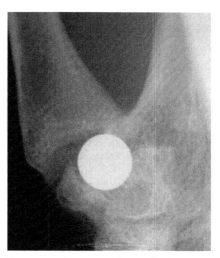

Fig. 20. Posteroanterior radiograph showing subsidence of Orthosphere prosthesis into the trapezium in a patient with symptoms of pain, weakness, and stiffness. (*From* Athwal GS, Chenkin J, King GJ, et al. Early failures with a spheric interposition arthroplasty of the thumb basal joint. J Hand Surg Am 2004;29(6): 1080–4; with permission.)

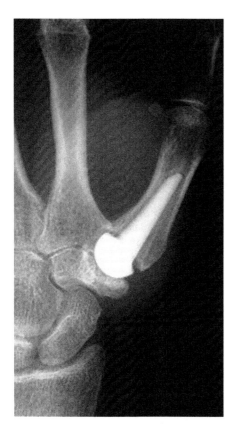

Fig. 19. A pyrolytic carbon hemiarthroplasty seen on posteroanterior radiograph at 17 months postoperatively. (*From* Martinez de Aragon JS, Moran SL, Rizzo M, et al. Early outcomes of pyrolytic carbon hemiarthroplasty for the treatment of trapezial-metacarpal arthritis. J Hand Surg Am 2009;34(2):205–12; with permission.)

and Associates, Flagstaff, Arizona) has also been tried with poor results.[96] Greenberg and associates[96] studied the outcomes of a Gore-Tex interpositional arthroplasty in 34 cases with 3.4 years of follow-up. Although there were good results in terms of pain relief and subjective outcomes, there was a high prevalence of radiographic osteolysis leading the investigators to recommend against the use of this material due to concerns of particulate synovitis (**Fig. 21**).

In contrast, an acellular dermal matrix allograft called Graftjacket (Wright Medical Technology) has been used as an interpositional arthroplasty with some favorable results. Adams and colleagues[12] described an arthroscopic technique for débridement and interposition with Graftjacket in the TM joint in patients with Eaton stages II and III disease (**Fig. 22**). This series reported generally good results with some symptom relief in all patients. 94% of patients were partially or completely satisfied, and 70% had no or only mild difficult in performing activities of daily living.

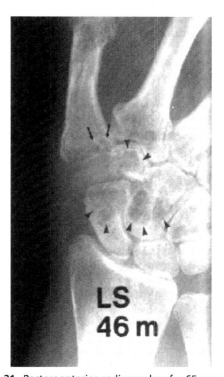

Fig. 21. Posteroanterior radiographs of a 65-year-old woman 46 months after a Gore-Tex interposition arthroplasty. The arrows highlight extensive osteolysis of the distal scaphoid, trapezium, capitate, hamate, and metacarpal base. (*From* Greenberg JA, Mosher JF Jr, Fatti JF. X-ray changes after expanded polytetrafluoroethylene (Gore-Tex) interpositional arthroplasty. Hand Surg Am 1997;22(4):658–63; with permission.)

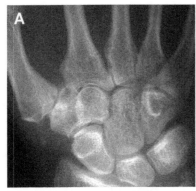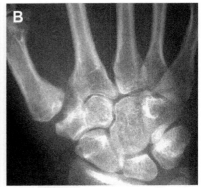

Fig. 22. Preoperative (*A*) and postoperative (*B*) posteroanterior radiographs of the TM joint after Graftjacket interposition, revealing increased TM joint space after interposition. (*From* Adams JE, Merten SM, Steinmann SP. Arthroscopic interposition arthroplasty of the first carpometacarpal joint. J Hand Surg Eur Vol 2007;32(3):268–74; with permission.)

SUMMARY

The optimal treatment of TM arthritis remains controversial, with no one technique proved superior. Prosthetic replacement arthroplasty of the trapezium has been available for approximately 5 decades. The most long-standing technology—silicone prosthetic trapezial spacers—may have a role in the treatment of low-demand rheumatoid patients, but overall outcomes have been poor and limited by silicone synovitis, implant failure, and loosening. Recent data on Artelon interpositional arthroplasty have shown inferior results compared with trapeziectomy and LRTI; given many case reports of foreign body reactions, the data lead to recommending against the use of this implant. Initial reports on metal total joint replacement of the TM joint were variable, with failures related to the significant forces across the base of the thumb, leading to loosening of the trapezial component in ball-and-socket designs and resurfacing implants devised in Europe and the United States. Recent studies, however, have shown that newer total joint prosthetic designs may have a better outcome than trapeziectomy with LRTI, at least in the short term. When compared with earlier studies, they were shown to have smaller rates of implant failure as well as superior pain relief, with better range of motion and grip strength.[59,61,63] Although pyrolytic carbon hemiarthroplasty has historically had higher complication rates than alternative procedures, this prosthesis may hold promise in the treatment of TM arthritis. Future research is needed to determine the long-term outcomes of the latest generation of pyrolytic carbon prostheses. Although the ideal implant may not be currently available today, the theoretic advantages for prosthetic trapezial arthroplasty should stimulate continued innovation in implant design and more rigorous prospective, controlled trials to better determine the role of any joint replacement of the TM joint.

REFERENCES

1. Peyron JG. Osteoarthritis. The epidemiologic viewpoint. Clin Orthop Relat Res 1986;213:13–9.
2. Davis TR, Brady O, Barton NJ, et al. Trapeziectomy alone, with tendon interposition or with ligament reconstruction? J Hand Surg Br 1997;22(6):689–94.
3. Davis TR, Brady O, Dias JJ. Excision of the trapezium for osteoarthritis of the trapeziometacarpal joint: a study of the benefit of ligament reconstruction or tendon interposition. J Hand Surg Am 2004;29(6):1069–77.
4. Taylor EJ, Sesari K, D'Arcy JC, et al. A comparison of fusion, trapeziectomy and silastic replacement for the treatment of osteoarthritis of the trapeziometacarpal joint. J Hand Surg Br 2005;30(1):45–4.
5. Eaton RG, Littler JW. Ligament reconstruction for the painful thumb carpometacarpal joint. J Bone Joint Surg Am 1973;55(8):1655–66.
6. Pellegrini VD Jr, Burton RI. Surgical management of basal joint arthritis of the thumb. Part I. Long-term results of silicone implant arthroplasty. J Hand Surg Am 1986;11(3):309–24.
7. Burton RI, Pellegrini VD Jr. Surgical management of basal joint arthritis of the thumb. Part II. Ligament reconstruction with tendon interposition arthroplasty. J Hand Surg Am 1986;11(3):324–32.
8. Weilby A. Tendon interposition arthroplasty of the first carpo-metacarpal joint. J Hand Surg Br 1988;13(4):421–5.
9. Heyworth BE, Jobin CM, Monica JT, et al. Long-term follow-up of basal joint resection arthroplasty of the thumb with transfer of the abductor pollicis brevis

origin to the flexor carpi radialis tendon. J Hand Surg Am 2009;34(6):1021–8.

10. De Smet L, Van Meir N, Verhoeven N, et al. Is there still a place for arthrodesis in the surgical treatment of basal joint osteoarthritis of the thumb? Acta Orthop Belg 2010;76(6):719–24.

11. Adams JE, Merten SM, Steinmann SP. Arthroscopic interposition arthroplasty of the first carpometacarpal joint. J Hand Surg Eur Vol 2007;32(3):268–74.

12. Menon J. Arthroscopic management of trapeziometacarpal joint arthritis of the thumb. Arthroscopy 1996;12(5):581–7.

13. Daroda S, Menvielle F, Cosentino R, et al. Arthroscopic total trapeziectomy. Tech Hand Up Extrem Surg 2010;14(4):259–62.

14. Adams JE, Steinmann SP, Culp RW. Bone-preserving arthroscopic options for treatment of thumb basilar joint arthritis. Hand Clin 2011;27(3): 355–9.

15. Badia A. Arthroscopic indications and technique for artelon interposition arthroplasty of the thumb trapeziometacarpal joint. Tech Hand Up Extrem Surg 2008;12(4):236–41.

16. Parker WL, Linscheid RL, Amadio PC. Long-term outcomes of first metacarpal extension osteotomy in the treatment of carpal-metacarpal osteoarthritis. J Hand Surg Am 2008;33(10):1737–43.

17. Futami T, Nakamura K, Shimajiri I. Osteotomy for trapeziometacarpal arthrosis. 4(1-6) year follow-up of 12 cases. Acta Orthop Scand 1992;63(4):462–4.

18. Wilson JN, Bossley CJ. Osteotomy in the treatment of osteoarthritis of the first carpometacarpal joint. J Bone Joint Surg Br 1983;65(2):179–81.

19. Tomaino MM. Treatment of Eaton stage I trapeziometacarpal disease. Ligament reconstruction or thumb metacarpal extension osteotomy? Hand Clin 2001; 17(2):197–205.

20. Swanson AB, deGoot Swanson G, Watermeier JJ. Trapezium implant arthroplasty. Long-term evaluation of 150 cases. J Hand Surg Am 1981;6(2): 125–41.

21. MacDermid JC, Roth JH, Rampersaud YR, et al. Trapezial arthroplasty with silicone rubber implantation for advanced osteoarthritis of the trapeziometacarpal joint of the thumb. Can J Surg 2003; 46(2):103–10.

22. Minamikawa Y, Peimer CA, Ogawa R, et al. In vivo experimental analysis of silicone implants on bone and soft tissue. J Hand Surg Am 1994;19(4):575–83.

23. Karlsson MK, Necking LE, Redlund-Johnell I. Foreign body reaction after modified silicone rubber arthroplasty of the first carpometacarpal joint. Scand J Plast Reconstr Surg Hand Surg 1992;26(1):101–3.

24. Creighton JJ Jr, Steichen JB, Strickland JW. Long-term evaluation of Silastic trapezial arthroplasty in patients with osteoarthritis. J Hand Surg Am 1991; 16(3):510–9.

25. Hirakawa K, Bauer TW, Culver JE, et al. Isolation and quantitation of debris particles around failed silicone orthopedic implants. J Hand Surg Am 1996;21(5): 819–27.

26. Naidu SH. Oxidation of silicone elastomer finger joints. J Hand Surg Am 2007;32(2):190–3.

27. Amadio PC, Millender LH, Smith RJ. Silicone spacer or tendon spacer for trapezium resection arthroplasty—comparison of results. J Hand Surg Am 1982;7(3):237–44.

28. Lanzetta M, Foucher G. A comparison of different surgical techniques in treating degenerative arthrosis of the carpometacarpal joint of the thumb. A retrospective study of 98 cases. J Hand Surg Br 1995; 20(1):105–10.

29. Lehmann O, Herren DB, Simmen BR. Comparison of tendon suspension-interposition and silicon spacers in the treatment of degenerative osteoarthritis of the base of the thumb. Ann Chir Main Memb Super 1998;17(1):25–30.

30. Lovell ME, Nuttall D, Trail IA, et al. A patient-reported comparison of trapeziectomy with Swanson Silastic implant or sling ligament reconstruction. J Hand Surg Br 1999;24(4):453–5.

31. Tagil M, Kopylov P. Swanson versus APL arthroplasty in the treatment of osteoarthritis of the trapeziometacarpal joint: a prospective and randomized study in 26 patients. J Hand Surg Br 2002;27(5): 452–6.

32. Bezwada HP, Webber JB. Questions regarding the Swanson silicone trapezium implant. J Bone Joint Surg Am 2002;84(5):872 [author reply: 872–3].

33. Minami A, Iwasaki N, Kutsumi K, et al. A long-term follow-up of silicone-rubber interposition arthroplasty for osteoarthritis of the thumb carpometacarpal joint. Hand Surg 2005;10(1):77–82.

34. Luria S, Waitayawinyu T, Nemecheck N, et al. Biomechanic analysis of trapeziectomy, ligament reconstruction with tendon interposition, and tie-in trapezium implant arthroplasty for thumb carpometacarpal arthritis: a cadaver study. J Hand Surg Am 2007;32(5):697–706.

35. Ashworth CR, Blatt G, Chuinard RG, et al. Silicone-rubber interposition arthroplasty of the carpometacarpal joint of the thumb. J Hand Surg Am 1977; 2(5):345–57.

36. Kessler FB, Epstein MJ, Culver JE Jr, et al. Proplast stabilized stemless trapezium implant. J Hand Surg Am 1984;9(2):227–31.

37. Gisselfalt K, Edberg B, Flodin P. Synthesis and properties of degradable poly(urethane urea)s to be used for ligament reconstructions. Biomacromolecules 2002;3(5):951–8.

38. Nilsson A, Liljensten E, Bergström C, et al. Results from a degradable TMC joint Spacer (Artelon) compared with tendon arthroplasty. J Hand Surg Am 2005;30(2):380–9.

39. Jorheim M, Isaxon I, Flondell M, et al. Short-term outcomes of trapeziometacarpal artelon implant compared with tendon suspension interposition arthroplasty for osteoarthritis: a matched cohort study. J Hand Surg Am 2009;34(8):1381–7.

40. Nilsson A, Wiig M, Alnehill H, et al. The Artelon CMC spacer compared with tendon interposition arthroplasty. Acta Orthop 2010;81(2):237–44.

41. Choung EW, Tan V. Foreign-body reaction to the Artelon CMC joint spacer: case report. J Hand Surg Am 2008;33(9):1617–20.

42. Giuffrida AY, Gyuricza C, Perino G, et al. Foreign body reaction to artelon spacer: case report. J Hand Surg Am 2009;34(8):1388–92.

43. Robinson PM, Muir LT. Foreign body reaction associated with Artelon: report of three cases. J Hand Surg Am 2011;36(1):116–20.

44. de la Caffinière JY, Aucouturier P. Trapezio-metacarpal arthroplasty by total prosthesis. Hand 1979; 11(1):41–6.

45. Chakrabarti AJ, Robinson AH, Gallagher P. De la Caffinière thumb carpometacarpal replacements. 93 cases at 6 to 16 years follow-up. J Hand Surg Br 1997;22(6):695–8.

46. Nicholas RM, Calderwood JW. De la Caffinière arthroplasty for basal thumb joint osteoarthritis. J Bone Joint Surg Br 1992;74(2):309–12.

47. Sondergaard L, Konradsen L, Rechnagel K. Long-term follow-up of the cemented Caffinière prosthesis for trapezio-metacarpal arthroplasty. J Hand Surg Br 1991;16(4):428–30.

48. van Cappelle HG, Elzenga P, van Horn JR. Long-term results and loosening analysis of de la Caffinière replacements of the trapeziometacarpal joint. J Hand Surg Am 1999;24(3):476–82.

49. Wachtl SW, Guggenheim PR, Sennwald GR. Cemented and non-cemented replacements of the trapeziometacarpal joint. J Bone Joint Surg Br 1998; 80(1):121–5.

50. August AC, Coupland RM, Sandifer JP. Short term review of the De la Caffinière trapeziometacarpal arthroplasty. J Hand Surg Br 1984;9(2):185–8.

51. De Smet L, Sioen W, Spaepen D, et al. Total joint arthroplasty for osteoarthritis of the thumb basal joint. Acta Orthop Belg 2004;70(1):19–24.

52. De Smet L, Sioen W, Spaepen D. Changes in key pinch strength after excision of the trapezium and total joint arthroplasty. J Hand Surg Br 2004;29(1): 40–1.

53. Ferrari B, Steffee AD. Trapeziometacarpal total joint replacement using the Steffee prosthesis. J Bone Joint Surg Am 1986;68(8):1177–84.

54. Hannula TT, Nahigian SH. A preliminary report: cementless trapeziometacarpal arthroplasty. J Hand Surg Am 1999;24(1):92–101.

55. Alnot JY, Beal D, Oberlin C, et al. GUEPAR total trapeziometacarpal prosthesis in the treatment of arthritis of the thumb. 36 case reports. Ann Chir Main Memb Super 1993;12(2):93–104 [in French].

56. Masmejean E, Alnot JY, Chantelot C, et al. Guepar anatomical trapeziometacarpal prosthesis. Chir Main 2003;22(1):30–6 [in French].

57. Masmejean E, Alnot JY, Beccari R. Surgical replacement of the thumb saddle joint with the GUEPAR prosthesis. Orthopade 2003;32(9):798–802 [in German].

58. Alnot JY, Muller GP. A retrospective review of 115 cases of surgically-treated trapeziometacarpal osteoarthritis. Rev Rhum Engl Ed 1998;65(2):95–108.

59. Lemoine S, Wavreille G, Alnot JY, et al. Second generation GUEPAR total arthroplasty of the thumb basal joint: 50 months follow-up in 84 cases. Orthop Traumatol Surg Res 2009;95(1):63–9.

60. Regnard PJ. Electra trapezio metacarpal prosthesis: results of the first 100 cases. J Hand Surg Br 2006; 31(6):621–8.

61. Ulrich-Vinther M, Puggaard H, Lange B. Prospective 1-year follow-up study comparing joint prosthesis with tendon interposition arthroplasty in treatment of trapeziometacarpal osteoarthritis. J Hand Surg Am 2008;33(8):1369–77.

62. Braun RM. Total joint replacement at the base of the thumb—preliminary report. J Hand Surg Am 1982; 7(3):245–51.

63. Badia A, Sambandam SN. Total joint arthroplasty in the treatment of advanced stages of thumb carpometacarpal joint osteoarthritis. J Hand Surg Am 2006;31(10):1605–14.

64. Ledoux P. Failure of total uncemented trapeziometacarpal prosthesis. A multicenter study. Ann Chir Main Memb Super 1997;16(3):215–21 [in French].

65. Cooney WP, Linscheid RL, Askew LJ. Total arthroplasty of the thumb trapeziometacarpal joint. Clin Orthop Relat Res 1987;220:35–45.

66. Uchiyama S, Cooney WP, Nieber G, et al. Biomechanical analysis of the trapeziometacarpal joint after surface replacement arthroplasty. J Hand Surg Am 1999;24(3):483–90.

67. Imaeda T, Cooney WP, Nieber GL, et al. Kinematics of the trapeziometacarpal joint: a biomechanical analysis comparing tendon interposition arthroplasty and total-joint arthroplasty. J Hand Surg Am 1996; 21(4):544–53.

68. Pérez-Úbeda MJ, García-López A, Marco Martinez F, et al. Results of the cemented SR trapeziometacarpal prosthesis in the treatment of thumb carpometacarpal osteoarthritis. J Hand Surg Am 2003;28(6):917–25.

69. van Rijn J, Gosens T. A cemented surface replacement prosthesis in the basal thumb joint. J Hand Surg Am 2010;35(4):572–9.

70. Swanson AB, de Groot Swanson G, DeHeer DH, et al. Carpal bone titanium implant arthroplasty. 10 Years' experience. Clin Orthop Relat Res 1997;(342):46–58.

71. Phaltankar PM, Magnussen PA. Hemiarthroplasty for trapeziometacarpal arthritis—a useful alternative? J Hand Surg Br 2003;28(1):80–5.
72. Naidu SH, Kulkarni N, Saunders M. Titanium basal joint arthroplasty: a finite element analysis and clinical study. J Hand Surg Am 2006;31(5):760–5.
73. Holland NB, Ruegsegger M, Marchant RE. Alkyl group dependence of the surface-induced assembly of nonionic disaccharide surfactants. Langmuir 1998;14:2790–5.
74. Hills BA, Monds MK. Enzymatic identification of the load bearing lubricant in the joint. Br J Rheumatol 1998;37(2):137–42.
75. Qiu Y, Qiu Y, Ruegsegger M, et al. Biomimetic engineering of non-adhesive glycocalyx-like surfaces using oligosaccharide surfactant polymers. Nature 1998;392:799–801.
76. Cook SD, Thomas KA, Kester MA. Wear characteristics of the canine acetabulum against different femoral prostheses. J Bone Joint Surg Br 1989;71:189–97.
77. Cook SD, Beckenbaugh RD, Redondo J, et al. Long-term follow-up of pyrolytic carbon metacarpophalangeal implants. J Bone Joint Surg Am 1999;81(5):635–48.
78. Wijk U, Wollmark M, Kopylov P, et al. Outcomes of proximal interphalangeal joint pyrocarbon implants. J Hand Surg Am 2010;35(1):38–43.
79. Nunez VA, Citron ND. Short-term results of the Ascension pyrolytic carbon metacarpophalangeal joint replacement arthroplasty for osteoarthritis. Chir Main 2005;24(3–4):161–4.
80. Parker W, Moran SL, Hormel KB, et al. Nonrheumatoid metacarpophalangeal joint arthritis. Unconstrained pyrolytic carbon implants: indications, technique, and outcomes. Hand Clin 2006;22(2):183–93.
81. Parker WL, Rizzo M, Moran SL, et al. Preliminary results of nonconstrained pyrolytic carbon arthroplasty for metacarpophalangeal joint arthritis. J Hand Surg Am 2007;32(10):1496–505.
82. Chung KC, Ram AN, Shauver MJ. Outcomes of pyrolytic carbon arthroplasty for the proximal interphalangeal joint. Plast Reconstr Surg 2009;123(5):1521–32.
83. Sweets TM, Stern PJ. Pyrolytic carbon resurfacing arthroplasty for osteoarthritis of the proximal interphalangeal joint of the finger. J Bone Joint Surg Am 2011;93(15):1417–25.
84. Sweets TM, Stern PJ. Proximal interphalangeal joint prosthetic arthroplasty. J Hand Surg Am 2010;35(7):1190–3.
85. Nunley RM, Boyer MI, Goldfarb CA. Pyrolytic carbon arthroplasty for posttraumatic arthritis of the proximal interphalangeal joint. J Hand Surg Am 2006;31(9):1468–74.
86. Tuttle HG, Stern PJ. Pyrolytic carbon proximal interphalangeal joint resurfacing arthroplasty. J Hand Surg Am 2006;31(6):930–9.
87. Bravo CJ, Rizzo M, Hormel KB, et al. Pyrolytic carbon proximal interphalangeal joint arthroplasty: results with minimum two-year follow-up evaluation. J Hand Surg Am 2007;32(1):1–11.
88. Bellemère P, Gaisne E, Loubersac T, et al. Pyrocardan implant: free pyrocarbon interposition for resurfacing trapeziometacarpal joint. Chir Main 2011;30:S28–35.
89. Stabler D. Pyrodisk trapezium replacement in Australian Hand Surgery Society Annual Scientific Meeting. Bunker Bay, Australia, March 19, 2011.
90. Ardouin L, Bellmére P. A five-year prospective outcome study of pi2 pyrocarbon arthroplasty for the treatment of thumb carpometacarpal joint osteoarthritis. Chir Main 2011;30:S11–7.
91. van Aaken J, Holzer N, Wehrli L. High failure rate treating CMC 1 osteoarthritis with PI2 pyrocarbon prosthesis. J Hand Surg Eur Vol 2011;36(Suppl 1):S45–56.
92. Martinez de Aragon JS, Moran SL, Rizzo M, et al. Early outcomes of pyrolytic carbon hemiarthroplasty for the treatment of trapezial-metacarpal arthritis. J Hand Surg Am 2009;34(2):205–12.
93. Colegate-Stone TJ, Garg S, Subramanian A, et al. Outcome analysis of trapezectomy with and without pyrocarbon interposition to treat primary arthrosis of the trapeziometacarpal joint. Hand Surg 2011;16(1):49–54.
94. Athwal GS, Chenkin J, King GJ, et al. Early failures with a spheric interposition arthroplasty of the thumb basal joint. J Hand Surg Am 2004;29(6):1080–4.
95. Adams BD, Pomerance J, Nguyen A, et al. Early outcome of spherical ceramic trapezial-metacarpal arthroplasty. J Hand Surg Am 2009;34(2):213–8.
96. Greenberg JA, Mosher JF Jr, Fatti JF. X-ray changes after expanded polytetrafluoroethylene (Gore-Tex) interpositional arthroplasty. J Hand Surg Am 1997;22(4):658–63.

Arthroplasty of the Scaphoid-Trapezium-Trapezoid and Carpometacarpal Joints

Alberto L. Lluch, MD, PhD[a],*, Marc Garcia-Elias, MD, PhD[a],
Alex B. Lluch, MD[a,b]

KEYWORDS

- STT arthritis • STT arthroplasty • CMC arthritis • CMC arthroplasty • Carpal boss

KEY POINTS

- Resection arthroplasty is an old, and yet reliable, solution for the isolated osteoarthritis (OA) of some joints of the hand.
- With low rate of complications, this technically undemanding option is ideal for the scapho-trapezial-trapezoidal joint OA, as well as for the OA of the carpometacarpal joints of the fingers.
- This paper reviews its indications, surgical, technique and results.

RESECTION ARTHROPLASTY OF THE SCAPHOID-TRAPEZIUM-TRAPEZOID JOINT

Most degenerative disorders of the wrist are secondary to alteration of relationships of the scaphoid bone, either from ligament injuries (scapho-lunate advanced collapse), pseudoarthrosis (scaphoid nonunion advanced collapse), or scaphoid malunions (scaphoid malunion advanced collapse). The only primary degenerative arthritis of the wrist is that of the scaphoid-trapezium-trapezoid (STT) joint. Its etiology is not completely understood, although multidirectional joint instability is the most likely cause, because most STT arthroses are seen in women, who also have a higher predisposition than men to develop trapezio-metacarpal (carpometacarpal [CMC]) and interphalangeal arthritis secondary to joint instability.[1–6]

The onset of symptoms is usually insidious and slowly progressive, although it can be precipitated by an injury such as a fall on the outstretched hand. Radiographic examination done at the time of consultation shows degenerative arthritis, proving that this may have remained asymptomatic for a long time. In some cases, the arthritis can be a radiographic finding during an examination done for other purposes.[7,8]

Some patients may have more pain at the radio-palmar aspect of the wrist, from synovitis of the flexor carpi radialis (FCR) tendon or ganglia originating from the scaphotrapezial capsule and migrating proximally along the tendon sheath.[9] The FCR tendon courses over the palmar surfaces of the scaphoid and trapezium in a separate fibro-osseous tunnel. Magnetic resonance imaging in patients with STT arthritis has demonstrated synovitis of the FCR, with partial or full-thickness tears, and ganglion formation.

Joint space narrowing, subchondral bone sclerosis, and peripheral hypertrophic spurring are observed. The most characteristic finding is shortening of the radial column of the carpus secondary to cartilage wear and bone collapse, also seen in cases of trapeziometacarpal joint arthritis. Most of the bone collapse is seen in the trapezium and trapezoid, causing an extended position of the scaphoid, best seen on lateral radiographs or computed tomography. Because the radial

The authors have nothing to disclose.
[a] Institut Kaplan for surgery of the Hand and Upper Extremity, Paseo Bonanova, 9, Barcelona 08022, Spain;
[b] Department of Orthopaedic Surgery, Hand Unit, University Hospital Vall d'Hebron, Paseo Vall d'Hebron, 119, Barcelona 08035, Spain
* Corresponding author. Institut Kaplan, Paseo Bonanova, 9, Barcelona 08022, Spain.
E-mail address: albertolluch@institut-kaplan.com

column of the carpus is shortened, the scaphoid will not be able to maintain the length of the central column, which progressively collapses, causing extension of the lunate and dorsal subluxation of the capitate (**Fig. 1**).

Indications

Patients with symptomatic, isolated, degenerative arthritis of the STT joint may benefit from conservative treatment.[1,2,6,10] This includes intra-articular injections of a synthetic corticosteroid (40 mg of triamcinolone acetonide) wrist immobilization in a removable splint, and an adequate program of hand therapy. Failing this, resection arthroplasty is recommended.

Fusing the STT joint is another alternative.[11] Unfortunately, morbidity associated with procedure is considerable.[12] Complications are frequent; most are a consequence of the scaphoid not being able adjust its position during radioulnar deviation. After fusion, the scaphoid becomes an unyielding prolongation of the distal row; therefore, in radial deviation, it impacts against the radius inducing early cartilage degeneration. Doubtless, if the midcarpal (MC) joint is stable, distal scaphoid excisional arthroplasty with or without interposition is more reliable, requires shorter immobilization time, and has fewer complications than a localized fusion.

Contraindications

Distal scaphoid resection arthroplasty is contraindicated when the STT degenerative arthritis is secondary to severe MC instability, a condition characterized by attenuation of the dorsal MC capsule and an excessively lax or underdeveloped dorsal intercarpal ligament.[13,14] To rule out this type of instability, the posterior drawer test is helpful.[15] Under fluoroscopic control, the distal row is forced passively toward the dorsum. If the capitate can be displaced beyond the dorsal limits of the scapholunate socket, the wrist has dorsal MC instability and requires a more aggressive procedure, such as STT arthrodesis, MC arthrodesis, or proximal row carpectomy. Treating global MC instability as if it was isolated STT arthritis could have devastating consequences: The attenuated dorsal MC capsule would not be able to prevent massive carpal collapse, with the proximal row rotating into severe dorsal intercalated segment instability (DISI) pattern of malalignment and the capitate subluxating dorsally.[14,16]

Operative Technique

Removal of the damaged distal articular surface of the scaphoid can be done arthroscopically.[17] Several publications have shown promising results with this technique.[18] In these authors' opinion, however, excising the bone is only a minimal part of the procedure. Rebalancing the capsule to prevent carpal malalignment is an essential part of this operation, and this can hardly be done arthroscopically. What follows is a description of

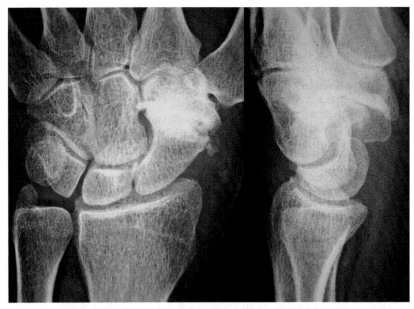

Fig. 1. Posterioranterior and lateral radiographs of a patient with severe degenerative arthritis of the STT joint, secondary to dorsal MC instability. Note in the lateral view how the lunate is abnormally extended and the capitate is translocated dorsally. Should this case be treated by distal scaphoid resection, a massive carpal collapse would follow.

the operative technique that we recommend for the treatment of isolated STT arthritis.[19]

A dorsolateral transverse incision over the anatomic snuff box, 1 cm distal to the radial styloid, is currently used to enter the STT joint. After carefully protecting the dorsal branches of the radial nerve, the deep fascia is released longitudinally. The radial artery is mobilized, its medial branches coagulated, and the main vessel retracted laterally. The prominent proximal edge of the trapezium and trapezoid bones are palpated and a transverse capsular incision is made just proximal to that prominence. This requires mobilizing the extensor pollicis longus tendon. At the level of the lateral border of the capitate, the capsular incision curves proximally along the scaphocapitate joint for about 5 mm. A similar oblique incision is done following the dorsolateral corner of the scaphoid. This creates a proximally based flap that is elevated to uncover the STT joint (**Fig. 2**A). To improve joint visibility, the dorsal osteophytes of the trapezium and trapezoid are removed with a rongeur.

The distal articular surface of the scaphoid is osteotomized with an oscillating saw. The plane of the osteotomy is important. The cut needs to be slightly inclined toward the palm, matching the inclination of the proximal articular facets of the trapezium and trapezoid bones. If the osteotomy is correct, when the wrist is placed in neutral position, the gap must have a cuboid configuration, with the 2 proximal and distal surfaces being parallel. The amount of bone to be resected is another important issue. If the resection is too small, painful impingement in radial deviation may follow; if it is too large, unnecessary instability may arise. In general, a resection of 3 to 5 mm, depending on the size of the hand, is adequate. Once the distal scaphoid has been removed, if there is an obvious scaphotrapezial impingement, some reshaping of the corners of the bone may be necessary.

It is important to acknowledge that this intervention solves 1 problem (a painful STT arthritis) at the expense of creating another problem (proximal row malalignment).[14,20] As stated, under normal loading conditions, the lunate is in equilibrium between the tendency of the scaphoid to rotate into flexion and the extension tendency of the triquetrum.[21] In theory, if scaphoid length decreases, the extension moment of the triquetrum is likely to predominate, and a DISI pattern of malalignment should appear. The degree of lunate malrotation, however, is not exactly proportional to the amount of bone resected. There are patients with large scaphoid resections who develop only mild DISI. Of course, these are the exceptions. In general, the shorter the scaphoid, the more the lunate will be pulled by the triquetrum into an extended position. To minimize the consequences of such an imbalanced situation, several strategies have been suggested.[22,23] What follows is a description of the 3 most commonly reported.

Dorsal MC capsulodesis

After a distal scaphoidectomy, excessive extension of the proximal row may be avoided by

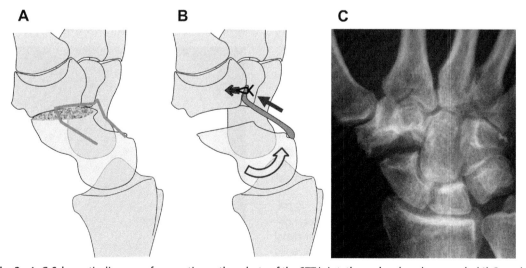

A   **B**   **C**

Fig. 2. *A–C*, Schematic diagram of a resection arthroplasty of the STT joint, through a dorsal approach. (*A*) Capsular incision used to create a proximally based capsular flap used to enter the joint. (*B*) The capsule is tightly reattached to the dorsum of the trapezium-trapezoid joint to prevent excessive extension malalignment of the proximal row. (*C*) Posterioranterior radiograph of a patient who underwent distal scaphoid resection arthroplasty without interposition 1 year previously. Cortical remodelling is evident at both sides of the excisional arthroplasty.

increasing the tightness of the dorsal MC capsule. Initially, this was done by creating a distally based capsular flap that was advanced onto the dorsal ridge of the scapholunate joint.[22] Unfortunately, adequate tensioning of the capsulodesis was not easily obtained, and a DISI pattern of malalignment often resulted. To overcome this problem, a reversed capsulodesis was recently suggested.[23] The proximally based capsular flap described is tightly sutured on the back of the trapezium and trapezoid by means of bone anchors (see **Fig. 2**B). This, together with a prolonged immobilization of 4 to 6 weeks, ensures acceptable results with minimal changes in carpal alignment (see **Fig. 2**C).

Palmar radiocarpal capsulodesis

Another alternative to prevent abnormal extension of the proximal row after a distal scaphoidectomy consists of increasing the tightness of the palmar radioscaphoid capsule.[23] This technique is particularly indicated in cases where STT arthritis coexists with a tenosynovitis of the FCR.[9] The STT joint is approached through a radioplamar incision centered on the scaphoid tuberosity. The FCR tendon is explored, and its inflamed tenosynovium excised. A distally based capsular flap is elevated to uncover the STT joint, and the damaged articular surface of the scaphoid is osteotomized and removed as described above. Using transosseous sutures, the most distal fibers of the radioscaphocapitate ligament are attached to the palmar edge of the osteotomized scaphoid. This creates a solid radioscaphoid tether that prevents the carpus from rotating into DISI. The wrist is immobilized for a period of 4 to 6 weeks, followed by proper hand therapy.

Resection and interposition arthroplasty

To avoid destabilizing the wrist after a distal scaphoidectomy, some authors have suggested resecting as much scaphoid as needed to alleviate symptoms, and filling the empty space with some sort of fibrous tissue, most often a rolled tendon.[19,23] In theory, by replacing the excised bone with a spacer, the scaphoid moment arm should be maintained, and the wrist should remain normally aligned. In practice, interposing fibrous material does not seem to prevent these wrists from developing secondary malalignment.

As an alternative, a pyrocarbon disk (STPI, Bioprofile-Tornier, Grenoble, France) has been developed to maintain the STT separation after distal scaphoidectomy (**Fig. 3**).[24–26] Certainly, a solid spacer is likely to be more effective is maintaining the carpal height than any fibrous interposition material (**Fig. 4**). Being completely unconstrained, however, the implant is free to move in the empty space, and the risk of dislocation is high.[23] To avoid

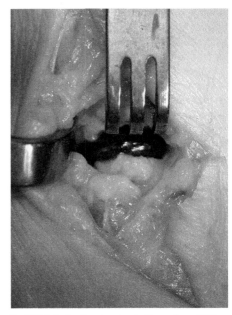

Fig. 3. Wrist just after implantation of an STPI spacer in the empty space created after resecting the distal scaphoid. In this case, a zig-zag skin incision was used. A more esthetical transverse skin incision is advocated presently.

implant subluxation, most authors advocate carefully closing the capsule, reinforcing the repair with local tissue, and immobilizing the joint for at least 4 weeks.[23] Other authors have suggested performing the entire procedure arthroscopically, with only a minimal capsular incision to insert the implant.[18]

Complications

As emphasized, the most serious complication of resecting the distal scaphoid is the development

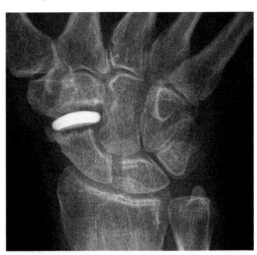

Fig. 4. Posterioranterior radiograph of a patient who underwent an STPI spacer for the treatment of an isolated degenerative STT arthritis.

of dorsal MC instability, characterized by severe rotation of the proximal row into DISI and dorsal capitate subluxation.[14,23] This is particularly prevalent among patients whose STT osteoarthritis is secondary to a chronic inflammatory process, such as chondrocalcinosis or rheumatoid arthritis.[27] Again, it is important to rule out, before surgery, the existence of a dorsal MC instability. Should this be the case, a partial fusion or a proximal row carpectomy is preferred.

Another possible complication, when a solid implant is used, is a dislocation of the spacer. Most often, the implant dislocates palmarly where it may impinge the FCR tendon, or radially where it may compress the sensory branches of the radial nerve. In both circumstances, removal of the implant may be required.

Results

A series of 21 wrists with an isolated STT arthritis were reviewed an average of 29 months (range, 12–61) after distal scaphoid resection arthroplasty.[19] The technique was found to reduce pain and to have less morbidity than what would be expected with an STT fusion. Wrist motion was not significantly different than before surgery. Grip was an average of 84% and pinch strength 92% of the contralateral side. Removal of the distal scaphoid, however, consistently resulted in an increased carpal misalignment, with 12 cases exhibiting substantial DISI pattern of misalignment, none of them symptomatic.

Similar clinical results, with a slightly lower incidence of residual carpal misalignment, have been reported with the use a pyrocarbon implant as spacer.[24–26] In this case, the problem is an 8% rate of implant dislocations.[23] Should a solution be found for these implants not to dislocate, that would be a step ahead in the solution of currently unresolved pathology.

ARTHROPLASTY OF THE II AND III CARPOMETACARPAL JOINTS

The proximal epiphyses of the finger metacarpals are solidly connected by stout and strong palmar and dorsal intermetacarpal ligaments (**Fig. 5**). The second metacarpal base has a sagittal notch, matching the convex shape of the distal articular surface of the trapezoid, and a dorso-ulnar extension, the so-called metacarpal styloid process, articulating with the corresponding distal facet of the capitate bone. The capitate has 2 distal articular surfaces: One wide, slightly concave, that articulates with the base of the third metacarpal; and a small facet in the radial corner of the joint for the styloid process of the second metacarpal. A

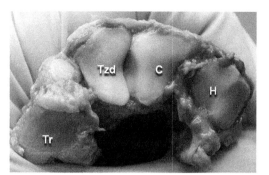

Fig. 5. Proximal view of the disarticulated CMC joints of a cadaver specimen, showing the distal articular surfaces of the trapezium (Tr), trapezoid (Tzd), capitate (C), and hamate (H) bones.

third small articulation for the fourth metacarpal may also exist, but it is not constant. The hamate articulates with the bases of the fourth and fifth metacarpals through 2 independent facets, separated by a sagittal prominence (see **Fig. 5**).

The CMC joints of the index and long fingers form a rigid structural unit. A tight arrangement of palmar and dorsal ligaments, supplemented by the distal insertions of the FCR and the extensor carpi radialis longus tendons, ensures such rigidity.[28,29] By contrast, the ligaments stabilizing the ulnar 2 CMC joints (dorsal, palmar, and intra-articular) are less stout, allowing 10° to 15° of flexion to the ring finger CMC joint, and 25° to 40° of flexion to the small finger CMC joint. This motion, produced by the hypothenar muscles and the extensor carpi ulnaris, allows control of the depth of the transverse metacarpal arch of the hand, and better grip adaptation to differently shaped objects.

Carpal Boss

Carpal bossing is a bony prominence at the CMC joints of the index and long fingers, described by Fiolle in 1931,[30] who called it *carpe bossu*. Several etiologies have been proposed, such as a periostitis from the pull of the extensor carpi radialis brevis tendon, an ossification secondary to rupture of the dorsal joint ligaments, an osteoarthritic osteophyte or the presence of an os styloideum (**Fig. 6**).

The presence of an os styloideum seems to be the most likely cause. This accessory ossification center is found in the dorsal quadrangular joint space formed by the trapezoid, the capitate and the bases of the second and third metacarpals (**Fig. 7**A). In addition to the normal 8 carpal bones, several accessory bones have also been observed. They usually disappear during fetal development, as a result of fusion or resorption.[31]

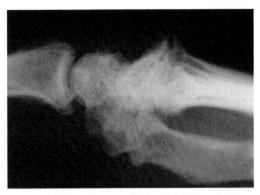

Fig. 6. Lateral radiograph of the wrist with a carpal boss.

The os styloideum corresponds to the styloid process of the third metacarpal.[32–34] In a study based on review a of 6000 radiographic examinations, Mangini[35] reported the os styloideum as the most frequent of all accessory carpal bones, followed by the paratrapezium, and then by the os centrale. The os centrale is located between the scaphoid, the trapezium and the capitate, usually uniting with the scaphoid toward the end of the second intrauterine month.[33]

If the accessory ossification center of the os styloideum remains, it generally attaches to the third metacarpal, and less frequently to the capitate, trapezoid, and second metacarpal (see **Fig. 7**B). In rare circumstances, it may remain as a separate ossicle.[36] During development, the cartilaginous anlage of bones forms around the 5th intrauterine week. At the site of future joint cavities a jelly-like substance appears and the cartilage becomes cleft into separate structures that will later form individual bones comprising the articulation.[37] The incidence of a persistent styloid bone is difficult to ascertain, and is best identified during anatomic dissections on cadavers. Thompson[36] reported 9 cases of a styloid bone in 564 dissected hands (1.6%), and Pfitzner[38] 46 styloid bones in 1456 dissected hands (3.1%).

Carpal boss seldom results from an isolated osteoarthritis of either the second CMC or third CMC. It is a more extensive problem involving the entire crossroads formed by the trapezoid, capitate, second, and third metacarpals. In most cases the problem predominates at the second CMC; in other cases it predominates at the third, but never is a purely isolated phenomenon.

The reason why only some carpal bosses are symptomatic is not completely clear but it seems likely that overuse, such as practicing sports like golf and racquet sports or trauma, will cause rupture of the fibrous union between the styloid bone and the capitate, as it usually incorporates as a bony fusion in the third metacarpal. Alemohamad and colleagues[39] reported that 10 of 87 pairs of wrists presented a carpal boss bilaterally (11%). The fact that most of symptomatic carpal bosses have been reported in the dominant hand makes one think that overuse may cause disruption of a fibrous carpal coalition. When an os styloideum is present, the normal dorsal CMMC joint ligaments are not fully developed, making this joint less stable and prone to painful instability during forceful activities of the hand.[28,29] Artz and Posch,[40] have observed a poorly formed bone-cartilage interface in most of their 57 operated cases, causing painful bone spurring after mechanical stress. A bone ossicle was removed in 3 cases.

Diagnosis is confirmed radiographically using a slightly supinated lateral radiograph of the wrist, called the "carpal boss view".[41] However with magnetic resonance imaging or, better yet with computed tomography, the osseous abnormality will be defined best (**Fig. 8**A, B).

In some cases, pain will be secondary to slipping of the extensor tendons of the index finger over the bony prominence on radial and ulnar deviation of the wrist.[42]

Resection Arthroplasty

Surgical treatment of carpal boss is only indicated in symptomatic cases, although sometimes we have also removed the osseous prominence for aesthetic purposes, particularly

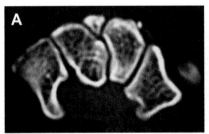
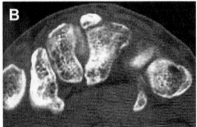

Fig. 7. (A) Computed tomography in the sagittal plane of an os styloideum. (B) Computed tomography in the sagittal plane of an os styloideum partially fused to the base of the third metacarpal.

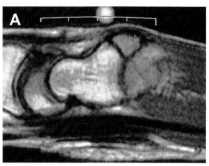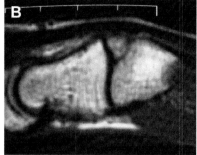

Fig. 8. (*A*) Computed tomography in the transverse plane showing an os styloideum between the bases of the second and third metacarpals. (*B*) Os styloideum as seen on a transverse plane of an magnetic resonance imaging.

in young women with very thin hands and large bony prominences.

Through a transverse 4 cm skin incision over the bony prominence, the extensor carpi radialis brevis tendon is identified. The tendon should then be dissected distally over the bony prominence being careful it is not completely detached from the base of the third metacarpal. After lifting and retracting the tendon toward the radial and ulnar sides, the osseous prominence is removed using a small bone rongeur and osteotomes.

If the osseous prominence is just removed to make it flush with the bony landmarks at the dorsum of the hand, recurrence of the prominence most likely will occur, as fibro-osseous tissue will form over the partially removed dorsal bones mimicking the old carpal boss in appearance, taking some time to flatten out completely (**Fig. 9**).[43–45] For of this reason, removal of bone and joint cartilage should be done until a moderate concave bone defect is created (**Fig. 10**).[46] However, a wide wedge excision of the bony prominence may lead to destabilization of the CMC joint, causing painful abnormal flexion mobility.[40,47,48] It has been recommended that wedge excision of the joint should not exceed 35% of the anteroposterior width of the CMC joint. Bone morphology, and the intact anterior and intercarpal ligaments will maintain joint stability. Excisions of more than 50% will cause abnormally increased flexion mobility of the joint.[49]

The wrist is immobilized with a plaster cast in slight flexion for about 10 days. Flexion of the wrist will prevent bowstringing of the ECRB tendon with secondary formation of scar tissue between the tendon and the denuded cortical bone. After removal of the cast the patient is allowed progressive unrestricted wrist mobility, except in those cases where the insertion of the ECRB tendon has been almost completely detached.

Complications

In cases in which painful flexion instability of the CMC joint occurred from excessive bone excision, an arthrodesis should be performed.

ARTHROPLASTY OF THE IV AND V CMC JOINTS

Although joint anatomy at the ulnar CMC joints can be quite variable, the convex base of the fifth metacarpal articulates with the concave ulnar facet of the hamate, while the base of the fourth metacarpal articulates with the radial facet of the hamate. These metacarpal bases also articulate with each other.

This articular anatomy, ligament structure and attachments, and the action of the tendons and muscles crossing both joints explain the greater motion of the ulnar side compared to index and long finger CMC joints. This mobility allows flattering and cupping of the hand with better adaptability and more effective grasp. Thus, activities such as handshaking, grasping a hammer or griping a racquet rely on the correct motion of the ulnar CMC joints.[50]

In contrast with the second and third CMC joints, the most common cause of arthritis in the ring and small finger is a sequelae of an intra-articular fracture of the metacarpal base with or without dislocation.[50] The initial lesion, frequently missed in high-energy trauma, usually results from striking an object with a clenched fist. This mechanism explains why it is predominant in men's dominant hand. Although specific patterns of injury were demonstrated in a cadaveric model,[51] the most frequent is a dorsal fracture dislocation, in which a variably sized palmar fragment remains in place. Easy to reduce, the lesion is difficult to hold and usually requires surgical treatment.

If left untreated, intra-articular fractures and fracture dislocations result in malunion that probably will end in CMC osteoarthritis. Surprisingly, good clinical results have been reported regardless of

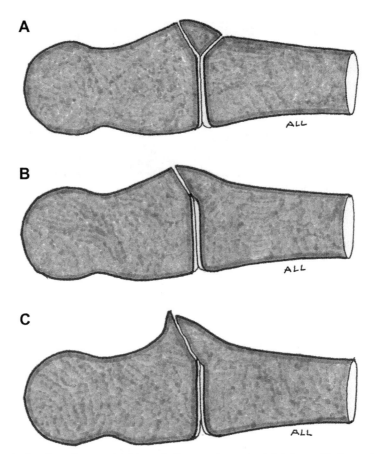

Fig. 9. (*A*) Schematic drawing of an os styloideum in the quadrangular joint formed between the trapezoid, the capitate and the bases of the second and third metacarpals. (*B*) Os styloideum fused to the base of the third metacarpal. (*C*) Degenerative arthritis at the underdeveloped joint between the os styloideum and the capitate, known as carpal boss.

intra-articular incongruity, subluxation or arthrosis after conservative treatment, or poor surgical reduction.[52,53] Thus, symptomatic posttraumatic arthritis at this level is less frequent than might be expected, as it happens after Bennet's fracture dislocation in the first CMC joint.

Treatment

When symptomatic, ring and small finger CMC osteoarthritis produces pain, weakness of grip, and secondary impairment. Nonoperative treatment should always be considered as the first option for these patients, including splinting, activity modification, and oral anti-inflammatory drugs. Despite being mentioned in many papers, intra-articular injections of corticosteroids are rarely useful, because these joints are quite narrow and difficult to inject.[54]

Patients with persistent pain and disability after conservative treatment require surgery. Some chronic cases, especially fracture dislocations in which the cartilage seem to be preserved may

benefit from open reduction and internal fixation even up to 4 or 6 months after the injury.

The most common treatment of symptomatic arthropathy of the ulnar CMC joints is arthrodesis of the involved metacarpal base to the hamate.[55] Arthrodesis eliminates articular pain and restores the length of the affected ray. However, bony fusion should be obtained and it has been said that, once the arthrodesis is obtained, the compensatory motion at the triquetohamate joint may predispose to degenerative changes at that level.[56] Moreover, in certain patients the sacrifice of motion at the ulnar CMC joints may also cause disability. For those cases, different types of arthroplasties have been proposed.

Silicone implant arthroplasty

Green and Kilgore in 1981[50] treated 2 cases of posttraumatic CMC osteoarthritis and 1 patient with juvenile rheumatoid arthritis, all of them with pain relief and good range of motion at an average follow-up of 20 months. Through a dorsal approach, a silicone toe implant was placed in the base of the

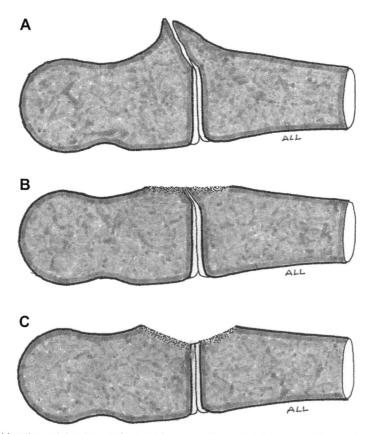

Fig. 10. (*A*) Carpal bossing originating at the joint between the os styloideum and the capitate bone. (*B*) Resection of the osseous prominence flush with the dorsal cortices of the carpal and metacarpal bones is not recommended, because recurrence will follow from scar and bone tissue overgrowth. (*C*) The recommended treatment is a wedge resection of the carpal boss until normal cartilage between the carpal bone and the base of the metacarpal is seen. To prevent joint instability, the resection should not exceed 35% of the CMC joint in the posterioranterior diameter.

fifth metacarpal. To avoid dislocation of the implant, they suggested using the smallest size implant and firmly closing the dorsal capsule. Apart from dislocation, silicone synovitis and implant rupture are potential complications of the procedure.

Partial resection arthroplasty

This procedure, proposed by Black and associates[55] for the treatment of osteoarthritis secondary to dorsal fracture dislocation, consists of resection of the dorsal impingement area. The joint, after the procedure, is based on the smaller but reduced palmar fragment with no attempt to reduce the dorsal subluxation. They reported no symptoms in 10 out of 13 cases 28 months after surgery, with 25° and 15° of mean motion at small and ring finger CMC joints. Grip strength became similar to the uninjured side.

Tendon interposition arthroplasty

Described in 1991 by Gainor and colleagues,[56] resection of the affected joint surface of the

metacarpal base, distal hamate, or both sides is followed by the interposition of a rolled tendon spacer (palmaris longus or a toe long extensor), supposed to act as a cushion between the 2 bones. The dorsal capsule is repaired, and the fifth metacarpal is pinned to the adjacent fourth metacarpal. After surgery the wrist is immobilized for 5 weeks. They treated 8 patients with this technique. All of them rated excellent or good functional and cosmetic results, and grip strength improved 30% at an average follow-up of 5 years. Metacarpal subsidence occurred in 6 patients, and egg cup remodeling and metaphyseal hypertrophy were present in 4 and 3 patients respectively.

Resection arthroplasty of the base of the fifth metacarpal associated with arthrodesis of the fourth and fifth metacarpals (stabilized arthroplasty)

In cases in which fifth CMC joint is affected but fourth CMC joint is not, an excision of the base of the fifth metacarpal is followed by an arthrodesis of the bases of the fourth and fifth metacarpals. By means of the resection arthroplasty, pain is eliminated. By means of the arthrodesis, mobility of the fifth metacarpal is obtained at the fourth CMC joint. Metacarpal length is thus restored and stability of the resection arthroplasty ensured. Nevertheless, mobility of the fourth CMC is approximately 50% of the fifth.

First described by Dubert in 1994, this procedure has several technical tips.[57,58] Done through a dorsal approach, the metacarpal base resection has to be parallel to the distal hamate articular surface (facing 30° palmarly) and not exceeding 10 mm, to maintain the insertion of extensor carpi ulnaris tendon. The length of the fused segment between the metacarpals must not be less than 1 cm, because otherwise it would not be strong enough, and no longer than 1.5 cm, to avoid extensive damage to the interosseous muscles. The intermetacarpal space should be filled with cancellous bone and the arthrodesis fixed with screws incorporating 4 cortices (**Fig. 11**). Bain and colleagues[59] modified the technique adding a dorsal periosteal/capsular flap as an interposition at the site of metacarpal base resection. They reported excellent results in 5 patients.

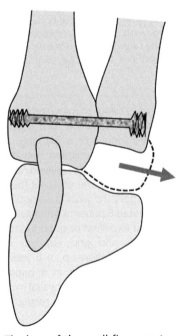

Fig. 11. The base of the small finger metacarpal and the distal metacarpal segment is arthrodesed to the ring finger metacarpal base. The arthrodesis is internally fixed with one screw incorporating four cortices. The intermetacarpal space can be filled a with a cancellous bone graft.

Complications

Apart from specific complications related to each technique mentioned, the most important complication of arthroplasty of the CMC joints of the ring and small fingers is persistence of pain. In such cases, secondary CMC arthrodesis should be the treatment of choice.

Another potential complication that has to be avoided is injury of the sensory branches of the ulnar nerve, which will always have to be protected during the dorsal approach of the ulnar CMC joints. In the uncommon situation that a resection of the distal hamate is necessary, care must be taken to avoid injury to the motor branch of the ulnar nerve, which runs palmarly just distal to the hook of hamate.

REFERENCES

1. Taleisnik J. Classification of carpal instability. In: Taleisnik J, editor. The wrist. New York: Churchill Livingstone; 1985. p. 235.
2. Linscheid RL, Lirette R, Dobyns JH. L'arthose dégénerative trapézienne. In: Saffar P, editor. La rhizarthrose. Paris: Expansion Scientifique Française; 1990. p. 185–93.
3. Sicre G, Laulan J, Rouleau B. Scaphotrapeziotrapezoid osteoarthritis after scaphotrapezial ligament injury. J Hand Surg Br 1997;22:189–90.
4. Pinto CL, Obermann WR, Deijkers RL. Nontraumatic multidirectional instability of the scaphotrapeziotrapezoid joint: a cause of scaphotrapeziotrapezoid osteoarthritis and static intercalated segment instability. J Hand Surg Am 2003;28:744–50.
5. Cooney WP. Commentary: multidirectional instability of the scaphotrapeziotrapezoidal joint. J Hand Surg Am 2003;28:751–2.
6. Van der Westhuizen J, Mennen U. A working classification for the management of scapho-trapezium-trapezoid osteoarthritis. Hand Surg 2010;15:203–10.
7. Crosby EB, Linscheid RL, Dobyns JH. Scapho-trapezial-trapezoidal arthrosis. J Hand Surg 1978;3:223–34.
8. White L, Clavijo J, Gilula LA, et al. Classification system for isolated arthritis of the scaphotrapeziotrapezoidal joint. Scand J Plast Reconstr Surg Hand Surg 2010;44:112–7.
9. Parellada AJ, Morrison WB, Reiter SB, et al. Flexor carpi radialis tendinopathy: spectrum of imaging findings and association with triscaphe arthritis. Skeletal Radiol 2006;35:572–8.
10. Wolf JM. Treatment of scapho-trapezio-trapezoid arthritis. Hand Clin 2008;24:301–6.
11. Wollstein R, Watson HK. Scaphotrapeziotrapezoid arthrodesis for arthritis. Hand Clin 2005;21:539–43.
12. Srinivasan VB, Matthews JP. Results of scaphotrapeziotrapezoid fusion for isolated idiopathic arthritis. J Hand Surg Br 1996;21:378–80.

13. Tay SC, Moran SL, Shin AY, et al. The clinical implications of scaphotrapezium-trapezoidal arthritis with associated carpal instability. J Hand Surg Am 2007;32:47–54.

14. Corbin C, Warwick D. Midcarpal instability after excision arthroplasty for scapho-trapezial-trapezoid (STT) arthritis. J Hand Surg Eur Vol 2009;34:537–8.

15. Park MJ. Normal anteroposterior laxity of the radiocarpal and MC joints. J Bone Joint Surg Br 2002; 84:73–6.

16. Linscheid RL, Dobyns JH, Beabout JM, et al. Traumatic instability of the wrist: diagnosis, classification and pathomechanics. J Bone Joint Surg Am 1972; 54:1612–32.

17. Bare J, Graham AJ, Tham SK. Scaphotrapezial joint arthroscopy: a palmar portal. J Hand Surg Am 2003; 28:605–9.

18. Mathoulin C, Darin F. Arthroscopic treatment of scaphotrapeziotrapezoid osteoarthritis. Hand Clin 2011; 27:319–22.

19. Garcia-Elias M, Lluch AL, Ferreres A, et al. Resection of the distal scaphoid for scaphotrapeziotrapezoid osteoarthritis. J Hand Surg Br 1999;24:448–52.

20. Garcia-Elias M. Partial excision of scaphoid: is it ever indicated? Hand Clin 2001;17:687–95.

21. Garcia-Elias M. Kinetic analysis of carpal stability during grip. Hand Clin 1997;13:151–8.

22. Garcia-Elias M, Lluch A, Saffar P. Distal scaphoid excision in scaphoid-trapezium-trapezoid arthritis. Tech Hand Up Extrem Surg 1999;3:169–73.

23. Garcia-Elias M. Excisional arthroplasty for scaphotrapeziotrapezoidal osteoarthritis. J Hand Surg Am 2011;36:516–20.

24. Pequignot JP, D'asnieres de Veigy L, Allieu Y. Arthroplasty for scapho-trapezio-trapezoidal arthrosis using a pyrolytic carbon implant. Preliminary results. Chir Main 2005;24:148–52.

25. Pegoli L, Zorli IP, Pivato G, et al. Scaphotrapeziotrapezoid joint arthritis: a pilot study of treatment with the scaphoid trapezium pyrocarbon implant. J Hand Surg Br 2006;31:569–73.

26. Low AK, Edmunds IA. Isolated scaphotrapeziotrapezoid osteoarthritis: preliminary results of treatment using a pyrocarbon implant. Hand Surg 2007;12:73–7.

27. Saffar P. Chondrocalcinosis of the wrist. J Hand Surg 2004;29:486–93.

28. Nakamura M, Patterson RM, Viegas SF. The ligament and skeletal anatomy of the second through fifth carpometacarpal joints and adjacent structures. J Hand Surg Am 2001;26:1016–29.

29. Nanno M, Buford WL Jr, Patterson RM, et al. Three-dimensional analysis of the ligamentous attachments of the second through fifth carpometacarpal joints. Clin Anat 2007;20:530–44.

30. Fiolle J. Le "carpe bossu". Bulletin et Mémoires de la Societé Nationale de Chirurgie 1931;57:1687–90.

31. Thilenius G. Untersuchungen über die morphologische Bedeutung accessorischer Elemente am menschlichen Carpus (und Tarsus). Morphologischer Arbeiten 1896;5:462–554.

32. Bassöe E, Bassöe HH. The styloid bone and carpe bossue disease. Am J Roentgenol Radium Ther Nucl Med 1955;74:886–8.

33. Kaplan EB. Functional and surgical anatomy of the hand. 2nd edition. Philadelphia: J.B. Lippincott Co; 1965. p. 123–6.

34. Köhler A, Zimmer EA. Grenzen des Normalen und Anfange des Pathologischen im Röntgenbild des Skeletts. 13th edition. Stuttgard (Germany): Georg Thieme Verlag; 1989. p. 80–103.

35. Mangini U. Os styloideum carpi. Arch Putti Chir Org Mov 1957;9.

36. Thompson A. The condition of the os styloideum as attached to the III metacarpal, to the magnum: to the trapezoid. J Anat 1894;28:64–6.

37. O'Rahilly R. A survey of carpal and tarsal anomalies. J Bone Joint Surg Am 1953;35:626.

38. Pfitzner W. Die morphologischen Elemente des menschlichen Handskelets. Z Morphol Anthropol 1900;2:77–157.

39. Alemohammad AM, Nakamura K, El-Sheneway M, et al. Incidence of carpal boss and osseous coalition: an anatomical study. J Hand Surg Am 2009; 34:1–6.

40. Artz TD, Posch JL. The carpometacarpal boss. J Bone Joint Surg Am 1973;55:747–52.

41. Conway WF, Destouet JM, Gilula LA, et al. The carpal boss: an overview of radiographic evaluation. Radiology 1985;156:29–31.

42. Kootstra G, Huffstadt AJ, Kauer JM. The styloid bone. A clinical and embryological study. Hand 1974;2:185–9.

43. Carter RM. Carpal boss: a commonly overlooked deformity of the carpus. J Bone Joint Surg 1941; 23:935–40.

44. Clarke AM, Wheen DJ, Visvanathan S, et al. The symptomatic carpal boss. Is simple excision enough? J Hand Surg Br 1999;24:591–5.

45. Park MJ, Namdari S, Weiss AP. The carpal boss: review of diagnosis and treatment. J Hand Surg Am 2008;33:446–9.

46. Fusi S, Watson HK, Cuono CB. The carpal boss. A 20-year review of operative management. J Hand Surg Br 1995;20:405–8.

47. Joseph RB, Linscheid RL, Dobyns JH, et al. Chronic sprains of the carpometacarpal joints. J Hand Surg 1981;6:172–80.

48. Citteur JM, Ritt MJ, Bos KE. Carpal boss: destabilization of the third carpometacarpal joint after wedge excision. J Hand Surg Br 1998;23:76–8.

49. Vermeulen GM, de With MC, Bleys RL, et al. Carpal boss: effect of wedge excision depth on third carpometacarpal joint stability. J Hand Surg Am 2009;34: 7–13.

50. Green WL, Kilgore ES. Treatment of fifth digit carpometacarpal arthritis with Silastic prosthesis. J Hand Surg 1981;6(5):510–4.

51. Yoshida R, Shah MA, Patterson RM, et al. Anatomy and pathomechanics of the ring and small fingers carpometacarpal joint injuries. J Hand Surg 2003; 28(6):1035–43.

52. Lundeen JM, Shin AY. Clinical results of intraarticular fractures of the base of the fifth metacarpal treated by closed reduction and cast immobilization. J Hand Surg Br 2000;25(3):258–61.

53. Kjaer-Petersen K, Jurik AG, Petersen LK. Intraarticular fractures at the base of the fifth metacarpal. A clinical and radiographical study of 64 cases. J Hand Surg Br 1992;17(2):144–7.

54. Hunt TR. Degenerative and post-traumatic arthritis affecting the carpometacarpal joints of the fingers. Hand Clin 2006;22(2):221–8.

55. Black DM, Watson KH, Vender MI. Arthroplasty of the ulnar carpometacarpal joints. J Hand Surg Am 1987;12:1071–4.

56. Gainor BJ, Stark HH, Ashworth CR, et al. Tendon arthroplasty of the fifth carpometacarpal joint for the treatment of posttraumatic arthritis. J Hand Surg Am 1991;16:520–4.

57. Dubert T. Stabilized arthroplasty of the 5th metacarpal bone. A therapeutic proposal for the treatment of old fracture-dislocations of the 5th metacarpal. Ann Chir Main 1994;13:363–5.

58. Dubert TP, Khalifa H. "Stabilized arthroplasty" for old fracture dislocations of the fifth carpometacarpal joint. Tech Hand Up Extrem Surg 2009;13:134–6.

59. Bain GI, Unni PM, Mehta JA, et al. Artrhodesis of ring finger and fifth metacarpal bases for small finger carpometacarpal joint arthritis. J Hand Surg Br 2004;29:449–52.

Proximal Row Carpectomy

Lindley B. Wall, MD[a], Peter J. Stern, MD[b],*

KEYWORDS

- Proximal row • Carpectomy • Kienbock's • Advanced collapse

KEY POINTS

- Proximal row carpectomy (PRC) is a motion-preserving surgical treatment for the degenerated wrist, specifically for scapholunate advanced collapse, scaphoid nonunion advanced collapse, chronic perilunate dislocations, and Kienbock's disease.
- The best candidates are older than 35 years with an intact capitate head and lunate facet of the distal radius.
- PRC provides satisfactory postoperative wrist range of motion and grip strength with few complications, especially when there is no capitolunate arthrosis.
- Postoperative progressive changes at the radiocapitate articulation have been documented, yet these changes tend to remain asymptomatic.

Proximal row carpectomy (PRC) is a motion-preserving surgical procedure utilized to treat degenerative conditions of the wrist. Although it is generally considered a salvage procedure and considerably alters wrist biomechanics,[1–5] it has been shown to reliably reduce pain and improve function.[6–19] PRC is a resection of the proximal carpal row and includes the triquetrum, lunate, and scaphoid bones, allowing the capitate to articulate with the lunate facet of the distal radius. The removal of pain producing articular surfaces and creation of the new radiocapitate articulation maintains wrist motion and can relieve pain.

BIOMECHANICS

Removal of the proximal carpal row greatly distorts the biomechanics of the wrist joint. Recent studies have investigated these changes.[1–6] Hawkins-Rivers and colleagues[1] analyzed 12 normal magnetic resonance images to assess the articular morphology of the capitate and lunate fossa, the new articulation created with a PRC. They determined that the radius of curvature of the capitate head is not congruent with the lunate fossa; it was found to be $37 \pm 10\%$ of the radius of curvature of the lunate fossa in the coronal plane and $57 \pm 10\%$ in the sagittal plane. Thus, it is clear that the radiocapitate articulation created by PRC is not anatomic and changes the native wrist biomechanics.

Zhu and colleagues[2] studied the biomechanical alteration created by a PRC by loading 6 cadaver specimens in 5 differing positions, before and after PRC, measuring pressure and contact area across the radiocarpal joint. They found a significant difference in the mean pressure seen after PRC ($P = .015$), a greater pressure seen in the wrist after PRC, with pressure greatest in the neutral position. The contact area was determined to decrease by 86% after PRC ($P<.001$). The contact area between the head of the capitate and radius was 0.33 cm^2, compared with 2.08 cm^2 for the radiolunate articulation. The increased pressure and decreased contact area seen in the PRC wrist were also reported by Tang and colleagues[3] utilizing loaded cadaveric specimens. These authors also found an increased pressure of 3.8 times the normal wrist and revealed a decrease in contact area, of 26% of the normal wrist, after

The authors have nothing to disclose.
a Washington University Orthopedics, 660 S. Euclid, Campus Box 8233, St Louis, MO 63110, USA; b Department of Orthopaedic Surgery, University of Cincinnati College of Medicine, PO Box 670212, Cincinnati, OH 45267-0212, USA
* Corresponding author.
E-mail address: sternpj@ucmail.uc.edu

hand.theclinics.com

PRC. Interestingly, however, in an earlier study by Hogan and colleagues[4] in 2004, although the pressure was seen to increase 57% of an intact wrist, similar to the previous studies, the authors found an increase in contact area by 37%. Perhaps difference in testing methods produced the conflicting results; however, all studies revealed that the PRC wrist undergoes a higher level of radiocarpal pressure and an altered contact area in comparison to a native wrist.

Not only does the wrist change in the degree of contact area and pressure seen at the distal radius articulation, the motion of the radiocapitate articulation differs from that of the intact wrist. Whereas Tang and colleagues[3] found both decreased contact pressure and contact area, as described, these authors also noted translational motion of the carpus after PRC. They found the capitate to translate at the radius articulation more that the native scaphoid. Hogan and colleagues[4] similarly found an increased amount of excursion in their study of 7 cadaveric wrists and postulated that this may help to explain the low incidence of degenerative changes in the new radiocapitate articulation. Along similar lines, Blankenhorn and colleagues[5] studied the kinematics of the PRC wrist utilizing cadaveric models. Their results also showed a translational component to capitate motion, similar to these studies. The authors found increased motion of the capitate compared with the intact wrist, where a combination of radiocarpal and midcarpal motions contribute to total wrist motion. This amount of wrist motion in the PRC wrist was concluded to be sufficient for activities of daily activities.

Interestingly, the change in load dissipation, consisting of both pressure and contact area alterations, and newly created articulation provides adequate motion and pain resolution clinically, as seen from clinical studies. It has been theorized that these good clinical results may stem not only from removing the degenerated native joint services, but also from the translational motion that results from the new capitate and radius articulation. The dissipation of load transmission is hypothesized to allow pain relief while maintaining motion.[3]

INDICATIONS

The primary indication for PRC includes arthrosis of the wrist. The most common etiologies include scapholunate advanced collapse (SLAC), scaphoid nonunion advanced collapse (SNAC), chronic perilunate injuries, and Kienbock's disease. A secondary indication for PRC includes the painful degenerated rheumatoid wrist. PRC can be performed in conjunction with wrist arthrodesis for end-stage arthritis or severe flexion contractures, placing the hand in a more functional position. The addition of the PRC limits the number of fusion sites and the extracted bones can be used for graft, limiting donor-site morbidity.[7]

All patients being considered for PRC should have failed nonoperative treatment and have chronic wrist pain that interferes with daily activities. The most common nonoperative treatment modalities include activity modification, anti-inflammatory medications, intra-articular corticosteroid injections, and immobilization. Additionally, other possible diagnoses must be ruled out, such as an inflammatory arthritic flare, tendinitis, fracture, or acute ligamentous injury. A third requirement for a conventional PRC is maintenance of the articular surface of the head of the capitate as well as the lunate facet of the distal radius. If there is radiographic narrowing of the capitolunate joint or degenerative changes, including sclerosis or cyst formation in the head of the capitate, the results of a PRC will be less satisfactory[9,10,12,20–22] and an alternative procedure, such as a total wrist arthrodesis or 4-corner arthrodesis should be considered.[18,23–26]

PREOPERATIVE EVALUATION

A thorough complete history of the involved extremity is required before surgery. Patient age and occupation must be noted, because these can influence choice of procedure. In addition, a history of trauma or chronic conditions and previous treatments should be documented.

Physical examination of the extremity is also necessary. This involves assessment of range of motion of the elbow, forearm, wrist, and digits. Wrist range of motion should include flexion, extension, and ulnar and radial deviation. Grip strength should be documented. Location of pain and the presence of dorsal–radial swelling should be noted. Finally, provocative tests reproducing the patient's symptoms should be documented.

Preoperative radiographic evaluation should include 3 views of the wrist: True posterioranterior and lateral views with the forearm in neutral rotation (**Fig. 1**A, B).[27] The authors have also observed that an additional clenched fist view can be useful in observing the amount of cartilage loss from the radioscaphoid articulation (**Fig. 1**C).

PREFERRED OPERATIVE TECHNIQUE

Regional or general anesthesia is utilized. The surgical limb is extended out onto a hand table and a tourniquet is used to create a bloodless field.

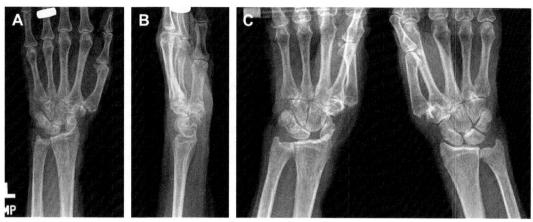

Fig. 1. (*A–C*) Preoperative radiographic studies: Posterioanterior, lateral, and clenched-fist views. (*A–C*), Preoperative views of the wrist of a 65-year-old female with a symptomatic chronic scapholunate advanced collapse injury. Note the widened scapholunate interval, flexed scaphoid, and degenerative changes at the radioscaphoid articulation.

A dorsal longitudinal incision is made sharply in line with the third metacarpal and running over Lister's tubercle (**Fig. 2**), extending from just distal of the carpus to about 1 cm proximal to Lister's tubercle, a total of 7 to 8 cm in length. The subcutaneous tissue is elevated from the extensor retinaculum and dorsal fascia with care taken not to divide the dorsal sensory branches of radial and ulnar nerves. The extensor retinaculum is divided sharply over the third compartment. The extensor pollicis longus tendon is transposed radially (**Fig. 3**). The posterior interosseus nerve is then identified and resected. We prefer a longitudinal capsular incision just radial to the extensor carpi radialis brevis to expose the carpus (**Fig. 4**). The fourth compartment is elevated subperiosteally in the ulnar direction, exposing the ulnar aspect of the distal radius and the lunotriquetral joint and triquetrum. Care must be taken to ensure protection of the dorsal radioulnar ligaments. Disruption of this structure could destabilize the distal radioulnar joint and result in postoperative wrist pain.

Before resection of the proximal carpal bones, the articular surface of the head of the capitate and the lunate facet of the radius must be inspected. If considerable degenerative changes are observed, the likelihood of a good result is decreased and soft-tissue interposition or wrist arthrodesis should be considered.

Once the proximal carpal row has been fully exposed, removal of the bones is addressed. A

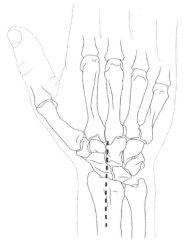

Fig. 2. Dorsal wrist incision, centered over Lister's tubercle. (*From* Stern PJ, Agabegi SS, Kiefhaber TR, et al. Proximal row carpectomy: surgical technique. J Bone Joint Surg Am 2005;86:166.)

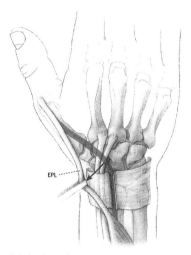

Fig. 3. Third dorsal compartment is incised and extensor pollicis longus tendon is transposed radially. (*From* Stern PJ, Agabegi SS, Kiefhaber TR, et al. Proximal row carpectomy: surgical technique. J Bone Joint Surg Am 2005;86:167.)

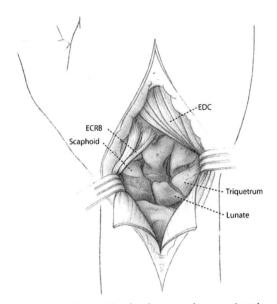

Fig. 4. Capsular incision has been made, exposing the proximal carpal row (triquetrum, lunate, and scaphoid) between the second and fourth dorsal compartments. ECD, extensor digitorum communis; ECRB, extensor carpi radialis brevis. (*From* Stern PJ, Agabegi SS, Kiefhaber TR, et al. Proximal row carpectomy: surgical technique. J Bone Joint Surg Am 2005;86:168.)

Knowles pin or large, threaded Steinmann pin is drilled into the scaphoid to facilitate its complete removal (**Fig. 5**). With sharp dissection around the scaphoid, particular attention must be paid to maintain integrity of the volar radioscaphocapitate ligament palmarly. This ligament provides stability to the wrist; its division can result in ulnar translation of the carpus. The radial artery, which overlies

the scaphotrapezialtrapezoid joint, is also in a position of danger and care must be taken not to damage it. The dissection continues and the entirety of the scaphoid is removed; however, and anecdotally from the senior author's experience, a retained scaphoid tubercle is not clinically problematic. After removal of the scaphoid, attention is turned to the lunate, which is removed by sharp dissection. Last, the triquetrum is removed. Removal of the proximal carpal bones en block should be attempted; however, if necessary, they may be removed piecemeal. Next the capsular incision is closed with a nonabsorbable 2-0 suture. Radiographs are then taken to confirm to resection and ensure that the head of the capitate is well-seated in the lunate facet of the distal radius (**Fig. 6**). In the authors' experience, experience it is not necessary to pin the radius to the carpus.

The extensor retinaculum is approximated with a 3-0 absorbable suture and the extensor pollicis longus is left radially transposed. A sterile dressing and palmar-based splint are applied, with wrist in 20° extension and metacarpophalangeal joints free.

POSTOPERATIVE CARE

At the time of first follow-up visit, the splint is removed and the wound inspected. The wrist is placed in a short arm cast. Finger motion is

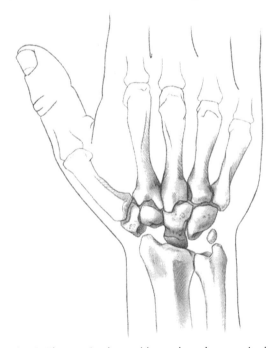

Fig. 6. The proximal carpal bones have been excised. The head of the capitate now articulates with the distal radius at the lunate fossa. (*From* Stern PJ, Agabegi SS, Kiefhaber TR, et al. Proximal row carpectomy: surgical technique. J Bone Joint Surg Am 2005;86:168.)

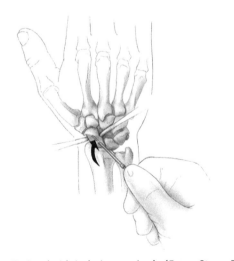

Fig. 5. Scaphoid is being excised. (*From* Stern PJ, Agabegi SS, Kiefhaber TR, et al. Proximal row carpectomy: surgical technique. J Bone Joint Surg Am 2005;86:168.)

encouraged while the wrist is continually immobilized for a total of 4 weeks. At 4 weeks postoperatively, a custom-made, volar-forearm–based wrist splint is fabricated and worn for an additional 3 weeks, coming out for gentle wrist range of motion exercises. Formal hand therapy is not necessarily required, but may help to reduce pain and encourage wrist motion. Passive range of motion is initiated at 6 weeks postoperatively. Full activities are allowed at 3 months postoperatively.

POSTOPERATIVE EVALUATION

The authors hold that PRC patients should be followed postoperatively for multiple years (**Figs. 7** and **8**). Patients should be monitored for any new onset of wrist pain; objective assessment and documentation of range of motion and grip are useful for detecting any possible symptomatic degeneration of the wrist. Radiographs should be obtained at the first or second postoperative office visit and then yearly to document any advancing disease of the radiocapitate space. That space can be classified based on the amount of narrowing: None, partial, or complete loss of space. This simple classification was proposed by Didonna and colleagues,[20] and is a very useful to monitor progression of radiocapitate degenerative changes.

OUTCOMES

The outcomes of PRC have been well-documented and there has been continued evidence of satisfactory results over the years, specifically satisfactory clinical function and postoperative pain relief.[8–20,28] Although first described by Stamm in 1944,[17] recent reports of long-term follow-up have been published. These long-term outcomes provide a perspective of clinical results beyond the immediate postoperative period and support the continued use of the PRC.[12,16,18,20,29,30]

Two studies in particular investigated the clinical outcomes with a minimum of 10-year follow-up of a mixed population of patients. In 2003, Jebson and colleagues[12] reported on the results of 18 patients who had undergone PRC for SLAC (7 patients), SNAC (10 patients), and chronic trans-scaphoid perilunate injury (1 patient) with an average follow-up of 13.1 years. Two patients, excluded from the study had undergone PRC and necessitated conversion to wrist arthrodesis at 28 and 40 months. The mean range of motion and grip strength of the remaining 18 patients, compared with the contralateral side, was 63% of motion and 83% of grip strength. Seventeen patients were satisfied. Radiographs revealed capitate head flattening in 6 patients; radiocapitate arthrosis was present in 17 patients, and moderate/severe in 4 patients. There was no correlation between the degenerative changes seen on radiographs and patient satisfaction or pain.

DiDonna and associates[20] published a similar study a year later and investigated the results of PRC in 22 wrists, in 21 patients, with a mean follow-up of 14 years. This study included a variety of diagnoses: SLAC in 9 patients, SNAC in 6, and Kienbock's disease in 7. Four patients in this series underwent wrist arthrodesis for continued pain at a mean of 7 years after PRC; all 4 patients were 35 years or younger at the time of the index procedure. The remaining patients had an average wrist range of motion of 71% of the contralateral side and grip strength of 91%. The average Disability of the Arm, Shoulder, and Hande (DASH) score was 9 for this group and 9 patients reported mildly or moderately painful wrists; no patient had a severely painful wrist. Radiographically, there was narrowing of the radiocapitate joint space in 7 patients and no visible space in 7 others. As shown in Jebson and colleagues'[12] study, the level of joint space loss did not correlate with symptoms. The authors concluded that, at a mean of 14 years postoperatively, outcomes are satisfactory for PRC in patients older than 35 years at the index PRC procedure. They also concluded that degenerative radiographic changes of the radiocapitate joint do not predict a poor outcome.

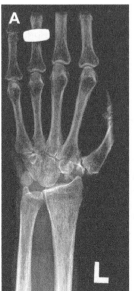
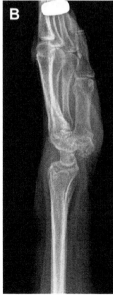

Fig. 7. (*A, B*) Postoperative views of the wrist 1.5 years after proximal row carpectomy.

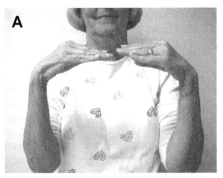 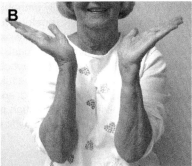

Fig. 8. (*A, B*) Clinical photographs of the patient's wrist motion at 1.5 years postoperatively; the left is the affected wrist.

Kienbock's Disease

Both of the mentioned studies provide long-term results of PRC for a mixed population of patients. Lumsden and colleagues[29] reported the outcomes with a minimum of 10-year follow-up for 13 patients with advanced Kienbock's disease. Lichtman's stage IIIA and IIIB in 12 of the 13 patients had good or excellent results. Compared with the contralateral side, wrist range of motion was 73% and grip strength was 92%. All patients had degenerative changes in the radiocapitate joint. Yet, as demonstrated by others, this did not correlate with painful symptoms.

Similarly, although slightly shorter in follow-up (average, 10 years; range, 4–17), Croog and Stern[30] also reported the outcomes for patients undergoing PRC for advanced Kienbock's disease. Twenty-three patients with a Lichtman's stage IIIA, IIIB, or IV were evaluated. Three patients—2 with stage IV disease—underwent wrist arthrodesis for continued symptoms after PRC at a mean of 23 months postoperatively. The other patients had a mean wrist range of motion of 78% of the contralateral side and grip strength of 87%. The mean DASH score was 12. Radiographically, there was radiocapitate joint degeneration in 16 patients with partial or complete loss of joint space in 14 patients. As seen with Lumsden and assocates'[29] study, the degeneration observed in the radiocapitate joint did not correlated with painful symptoms. The authors also noted that particular caution should be given to patients with stage IV Kienbock's because of the increased risk of continued pain necessitating conversion to wrist arthrodesis after PRC.

Chronic Perilunate Injury

Chronic perilunate injury is another cause of degenerative wrist disease. Rettig and Raskin,[16] in 1999, reported the results of 12 patients in this subgroup treated with PRC, with an average follow-up of 40 months. These patients had a chronic stage III or IV perilunate injury and did not undergo acute or complete treatment for 1 of 3 reasons: Medical treatment was not sought, the injury was unrecognized, or an incomplete reduction was obtained. All patients underwent median nerve decompression at the time of PRC. Surgery was performed through a combined dorsal/palmar approach, with temporary K-wire fixation (a technique we no longer recommend). Wrist range of motion averaged 80°, with no comparison with the contralateral side, and grip strength was 80% of the contralateral side. All patients reported improvement in wrist pain and in median nerve symptoms; only 3 had mild occasional pain and 3 had numbness in the median nerve distribution at follow-up. Radiographic follow-up revealed maintained carpal alignment, with 1 patient developing radiocapitate degenerative changes. Of note, this patient had documented capitate degeneration at the index procedure. The authors concluded by recommending PRC for chronic perilunate injuries and they noted improvement in both painful symptoms and function.

PRC in Acute Injury

PRC is conventionally performed for chronic pathology of the wrist; however, it has also been described for treatment of acute wrist injuries.[15,31–35] PRC has been reported with hand replantations,[32] severe open wrist injuries with significant bone loss,[31] and various other clinical situations.[15,33] Della Santa and colleagues[34] performed a comparative study investigating the results of the acute (0–21 days after injury) use of PRC for irreducible or nonsuccessfully reconstructed perilunate injuries versus elective PRC for chronic conditions. Twelve patients were included in the study, 6 emergent and 6 elective PRCs. The authors found that all the emergency case patients were satisfied with their postoperative outcomes at a mean follow-up of 3 years, whereas only 50% of the elective surgery patients were satisfied (P = .046). Wrist motion was similar, at 54% and 66% of the contralateral side in the emergent and elective groups, respectively. Grip strength was greater in the emergent group, 71% versus 59% of the contralateral side (P = .047). Radiographically, 2 patients in the emergent group revealed radiocapitate changes (both had had an ipsilateral distal radius fracture at the time of injury), whereas 5 of 6 of the elective patients had degenerative changes. Mayo wrist score revealed no poor results with emergent surgery and 3 poor results in the elective group. This study provided evidence that emergent use of PRC is well tolerated. However, it is necessary to follow these patients over time to monitor for development of any progressive symptoms in the long term before recommending the acute use of PRC as a standard treatment option in this population.

PRC can also be used for acute ligamentous wrist injury. However, when PRC is used for scapholunate dissociation without radiographic degenerative changes, the results are not as favorable as those seen with Kienbock's and chronic perilunate injuries, even in the short term. Elfar and Stern[35] reported results of 31 patients who underwent PRC for static scapholunate dissociation without evidence of degenerative changes with a follow-up of an average of 20 months (range, 6–81). They found that wrist range of motion was 54% of the contralateral side and grip strength was 56%, results that are much poorer than those previously published for PRC. In addition, 48% of the patients reported moderate or severe pain and 4 patients failed PRC, necessitating wrist arthrodesis. The authors concluded that PRC is not a good treatment option for patients with static scapholunate dissociation without degenerative changes.

Wrist Arthrodesis

Although the literature reports satisfactory outcomes of PRC, there are some patients who continue to have wrist pain after PRC. The salvage procedure for PRC is a wrist arthrodesis,[18,23–26] which eliminates the remaining motion of the wrist and removes possible painful articulations. At a follow-up of longer than 10 years, the rate of wrist arthrodesis for PRC ranged from 10% to 18%.[12,20]

PRC VERSUS 4-CORNER ARTHRODESIS

PRC is not the only motion-preserving treatment for degenerative disease of the wrist; 4-corner arthrodesis is an alternative treatment option. The advantage of PRC is that it is technically less

strenuous, allows for early mobilization, and is not dependent on bony union. In contrast, 4-corner arthrodesis maintains carpal height, preserves physiologic motion by utilizing the radiolunate and ulnocarpal joints, and creates a more stable wrist joint. Controversy continues to exist about which of these 2 procedures results in most satisfactory clinical outcome for the degenerative, painful wrist.

Numerous studies have documented good results for both procedures, although few have compared PRC directly with 4-corner arthrodesis.[8,19,28,36] Comparing 9 patients after 4-corner fusion and 15 after PRC, Tomaino and colleagues[19] found that, although strength was similar, wrist range of motion was superior in the PRC group. However, 20% of the PRC group was not satisfied with the postoperative outcome. The authors concluded by recommending PRC in the absence of arthrosis on the head of the capitate.

Wyrick and colleagues[28] investigated a larger group of patients with SLAC wrist, 17 treated with 4-corner fusion and 10 with PRC, with follow-up of longer than 1 year. The authors found better wrist range of motion with PRC, 64% versus 47% of the uninvolved side, compared with 4-corner fusion. Similarly, the results revealed greater grip strength with PRC, 94% versus 74% of the contralateral side. There were also 5 failures in the 4-corner group, all resulting in wrist arthrodesis for continued pain. These authors[28] recommended PRC for motion-preserving treatment for degenerative SLAC wrist, with the caveat that the patients do not have degenerative changes at the capitolunate articulation.

In another study, Cohen and Kozin,[8] reported, from 2 separate institutions, on 2 cohorts of patients who underwent PRC or 4-corner arthrodesis for SLAC wrist. There were 19 patients in each group and all patients were followed for longer than 1 year. In this study, there was no difference in flexion–extension arc of motion—62% of the contralateral side in the PRC group versus 58% in the 4-corner group. In addition, grip strength was similar: 71% in the PRC group and 79% in the 4-corner group. Pain relief and postoperative satisfaction were similar between the 2 groups. The only difference was that the 4-corner group had a greater degree of radioulnar deviation than did the PRC group. The authors recommended both procedures as motion-sparing options for degenerative SLAC wrist based on short-term follow-up.

More recently, in a retrospective study by Vanhove and colleagues,[36] 30 patients were investigated at a mean follow-up of 3.5 months. The authors found that there was an increased complication rate with the 4-corner arthrodesis, including carpal tunnel syndrome, postoperatively. In addition, they noted an increased hospital stay and time off work for the 4-corner arthrodesis. Thus, the authors recommended PRC over 4-corner arthrodesis in patients with a well-maintained capitate head articular surface.

These studies sought to address the controversy of superiority of PRC or 4-corner arthrodesis and the results show a trend toward PRC when capitate head articular surface is maintained. Nevertheless, there is a need for a prospective, randomized trial to better delineate the specific indications, advantages, and outcomes for each procedure.

ALTERNATIVE TECHNIQUES
Arthroscopy

With the advance of minimally invasive operative techniques and use of wrist arthroscopy, it is not surprising that such techniques have been utilized for the PRC.[37–39] This approach theoretically can decrease the morbidity of open surgery and accelerate the postoperative recovery. Recently, Weiss and colleagues[39] reported their technique and outcomes for arthroscopic PRC. They reported the results on 16 patients, average age 56 years, treated with arthroscopic PRC with a minimum of 1 year of follow-up. The primary pathology of the study population was SLAC wrist. Wrist arthroscopy utilized the 3–4, 4–5, 6R, 6U, and midcarpal radial and ulnar portals. After the diagnostic arthroscopy was completed, the PRC was performed through the midcarpal portals by use of a 4.0-mm bur. No complications were noted and no surgery had to be converted to an open procedure. Postoperatively, wrist flexion–extension arc was 80% of the contralateral side and grip strength was 81%. The mean DASH was 21 and all patients reported being satisfied with the surgery.

Arthroscopic PRC seems to produce results similar to the traditional open technique with a theoretical decrease in morbidity and faster rehabilitation. However, further scrutiny of this technique is necessary to provide evidence to this fact. At this time, open PRC remains our technique of choice.

Interposition Arthroplasty and Capitate Resurfacing

Postoperative wrist motion after PRC is through the radiocapitate articulation; thus, patients with degenerative changes on the capitate head have less satisfactory outcomes.[9,10,12,20–22] An attempt to improve this articulation when arthrosis is present has been proposed by utilizing soft-tissue interposition arthroplasty (**Figs. 9–12**)[40–43]

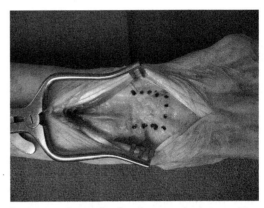

Fig. 9. Dorsal capsular flap for capsular interposition. The flap is marked out, 2–3 cm wide and proximally based. It must be noted that the capsule may be attenuated in SLAC and SNAC deformities.

or capitate resurfacing.[44] Eaton[45] described the technique of soft-tissue interposition arthroplasty in 1997. Approximately 2 decades later, the outcome of soft-tissue interposition has been reported. Kwon and colleagues[42] retrospectively reviewed the results of 8 patients who underwent capsular interposition with PRC. All patients had severe degenerative changes on the capitate and/or lunate facet; therefore, this procedure was performed to avoid wrist arthrodesis. Although wrist motion and grip strength were similar to preoperative levels at an average of 41 months of follow-up, all patients reported considerable improvement. Three patients had progressive radiographic changes at the radiocapitate joint, although their results were not different from those who had no progression. This approach for treatment of severe capitate head degeneration can also be coupled with capitate head resection, as reported by Placzek and

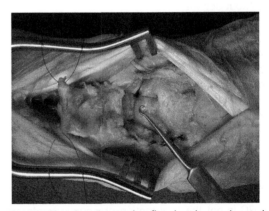

Fig. 10. The dorsal capsular flap has been elevated and reflected proximally, exposing the underlying carpus. The hook is placed over the head of the capitate for retraction.

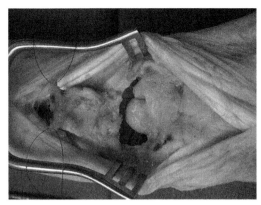

Fig. 11. The proximal carpal row has been removed.

colleagues,[40] with successful pain relief in expected in 75% of patients.

To investigate the biomechanical effects of soft-tissue interposition with PRC, Nanavati and colleagues[41] performed a study of PRC with interposition of lateral meniscal allograft in 6 cadaver specimens. They found the meniscal interposition restores the pressures and the contact area in the radiocarpal joint to level observed in the intact wrist. At present, we consider this technique investigational.

Another approach to severe degeneration of the capitate, as proposed by Tang and Imbriglia,[44] is osteochondral resurfacing of the capitate head at the time of PRC. The technique utilizes an osteochondral graft from one of the resected carpal bones with normal articular cartilage. The results of 8 patients were reported at 18 months of follow-up. Seven of the 8 patients reported no or mild pain; wrist range of motion was 66% of the contralateral side, and grip strength was 71%. Radiographically, 75% of patients had mild to no progressive degenerative changes and magnetic resonance imaging follow-up performed in 1

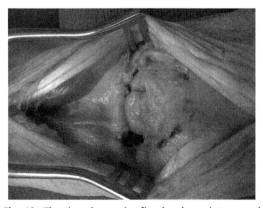

Fig. 12. The dorsal capsular flap has been interposed between the lunate fossa and the head of the capitate and sutured into the palmar capsule.

patient revealed graft incorporation. These results are similar to the results of standard PRC. With additional studies and increased follow-up, this technique could provide an alternative satisfactory treatment option for patients with degenerative changes of the proximal capitate for whom PRC could have questionable results.

SUMMARY

PRC is a motion-preserving operative treatment for the degenerated wrist, specifically for SLAC, SNAC, chronic perilunate dislocations, and Kienbock's disease. It seems that the best candidates are older than 35 years with intact capitate head and lunate facet of the distal radius. PRC may also have a role in the treatment of specific acute wrist injuries. PRC provides satisfactory postoperative wrist range of motion and grip strength with few complications, especially when there is no capitolunate arthrosis. Evidence of postoperative progressive changes at the radiocapitate articulation has been documented, yet these changes tend to remain asymptomatic.

REFERENCES

1. Hawkins-Rivers S, Budoff JE, Ismaily SK, et al. MRI study of the capitate, lunate, and lunate fossa with relevance to proximal row carpectomy. J Hand Surg Am 2008;33:841–9.
2. Zhu YL, Xu YQ, Ding J, et al. Biomechanics of the wrist after proximal row carpectomy in cadavers. J Hand Surg Eur 2010;35:43–5.
3. Tang P, Gauvin J, Muriuki M, et al. Comparison of the "contact biomechanics" of the intact and proximal row carpectomy wrist. J Hand Surg Am 2009;34:660–70.
4. Hogan CJ, McKay PL, Degnan GG. Changes in radiocarpal loading characteristics after proximal row carpectomy. J Hand Surg Am 2004;29:1109–13.
5. Blankenhorn BD, Pfaeffle HJ, Tang P, et al. Carpal kinematics after proximal row carpectomy. J Hand Surg Am 2007;32:37–46.
6. Sobczak S, Rotsaert P, Vancabeke M, et al. Effects of proximal row carpectomy on wrist biomechanics: a cadaveric study. Clin Biomech 2011;26:718–24.
7. Hartigan BJ, Nagle DJ, Foley MJ. Wrist arthrodesis with excision of the proximal carpal bones using the AO/ASIF wrist fusion plate and local bone graft. J Hand Surg Br 2001;26:247–51.
8. Cohen MS, Kozin SH. Degenerative arthritis of the wrist: proximal row carpectomy versus scaphoid excision and four-corner arthrodesis. J Hand Surg Am 2001;26:94–104.
9. Crabbe WA. Excision of the proximal row of the carpus. J Bone Joint Surg Br 1964;46:708–11.

10. Culp RW, McGuigan FX, Turner MA, et al. Proximal row carpectomy: a multicenter study. J Hand Surg Am 1993;18:19–25.
11. Ferlic DC, Clayton ML, Mills MF. Proximal row carpectomy: review of rheumatoid and nonrheumatoid wrists. J Hand Surg Am 1991;16:420–4.
12. Jebson PJ, Hayes EP, Engber WD. Proximal row carpectomy: a minimum 10-year follow-up study. J Hand Surg Am 2003;28:561–9.
13. Jorgensen EC. Proximal-row carpectomy. An end-result study of twenty-two cases. J Bone Joint Surg Am 1969;51:1104–11.
14. Lin HH, Stern PJ. 'Salvage' procedures in the treatment of Kienbock's disease. Proximal row carpectomy and total wrist arthrodesis. Hand Clin 1993;9:521–6.
15. Neviaser RJ. Proximal row carpectomy for posttraumatic disorders of the carpus. J Hand Surg 1983;8:301–5.
16. Rettig ME, Raskin KB. Long-term assessment of proximal row carpectomy for chronic perilunate dislocations. J Hand Surg Am 1999;24:1231–6.
17. Stamm TT. Excision of the proximal row of the carpus. Proc R Soc Med 1944;38:74–5.
18. Tomaino MM, Delsignore J, Burton RI. Long-term results following proximal row carpectomy. J Hand Surg Am 1994;19:694–703.
19. Tomaino MM, Miller RJ, Cole I, et al. Scapholunate advanced collapse wrist: proximal row carpectomy or limited wrist arthrodesis with scaphoid excision? J Hand Surg Am 1994;19:134–42.
20. DiDonna ML, Kiefhaber TR, Stern PJ. Proximal row carpectomy: study with a minimum of ten years of follow-up. J Bone Joint Surg Am 2004;86:2359–65.
21. Inglis AE, Jones EC. Proximal-row carpectomy for diseases of the proximal row. J Bone Joint Surg Am 1977;59:460–3.
22. Imbriglia JE, Broudy AS, Hagberg WC, et al. Proximal row carpectomy: clinical evaluation. J Hand Surg Am 1990;15:426–30.
23. De Smet L, Robijns F, Degreef I. Outcome of proximal row carpectomy. Scand J Plast Reconstr Surg Hand Surg 2006;40:302–6.
24. Nagelvoort RW, Kon M, Schuurman AH. Proximal row carpectomy: a worthwhile salvage procedure. Scand J Plast Reconstr Surg Hand Surg 2002;36:289–99.
25. Nakamura R, Horii E, Watanabe K, et al. Proximal row carpectomy versus limited wrist arthrodesis for advanced Kienbock's disease. J Hand Surg Br 1998;23:741–5.
26. Streich NA, Martini AK, Daecke W. Proximal row carpectomy: an adequate procedure in carpal collapse. Int Orthop 2008;32:85–9.
27. Chhabra AB, Miller CD, Wall L. Imaging. In: Hammert WC, Calfee RP, Bozentka DJ, et al, editors. Manual of hand surgery. Philadelphia: Lippincott Williams &Wilkins; 2010. p. 7–28.
28. Wyrick JD, Stern PJ, Kiefhaber TR. Motion-preserving procedures in the treatment of scapholunate advanced collapse wrist: proximal row carpectomy versus four-corner arthrodesis. J Hand Surg Am 1995;20:965–70.
29. Lumsden BC, Stone A, Engber WD. Treatment of advanced-stage Kienbock's disease with proximal row carpectomy: an average 15-year follow-up. J Hand Surg Am 2008;33:493–502.
30. Croog AS, Stern PJ. Proximal row carpectomy for advanced Kienbock's disease: average 10-year follow-up. J Hand Surg Am 2008;33:1122–30.
31. Marin-Braun F. Emergency proximal row carpectomy. Ann Chir Main 1992;11:283–4.
32. Meyer VE. Hand amputations proximal but close to the wrist joint: prime candidates for reattachment (long-term functional results). J Hand Surg Am 1985;10:989–91.
33. Van Kooten EO, Coster E, Segers MJ, et al. Review article. Early proximal row carpectomy. Injury 2005;36:1226–32.
34. Della Santa DR, Sennwald GR, Mathys L, et al. Proximal row carpectomy in emergency. Chir Main 2010;29:224–30.
35. Elfar JC, Stern PJ. Proximal row carpectomy for scapholunate dissociation. J Hand Surg Eur 2011;36:111–5.
36. Vanhove W, De Vil J, Van Seymortier P, et al. Proximal row carpectomy versus four-corner arthrodesis as a treatment for SLAC (scapholunate advanced collapse) wrist. J Hand Surg Eur 2008;33:118–25.
37. Culp RW, Osterman AL, Talsania JS. Arthroscopic proximal row carpectomy. Tech Hand Up Extrem Surg 1997;1A:116–9.
38. Roth JH, Poehling GG. Arthroscopic "-ectomy" surgery of the wrist. Arthroscopy 1990;6A:141–7.
39. Weiss ND, Molina RA, Gwin S. Arthroscopic proximal row carpectomy. J Hand Surg Am 2011;36:577–82.
40. Placzek JD, Boyer MI, Raaii F, et al. Proximal row carpectomy with capitate resection and capsular interposition for treatment of scapholunate advanced collapse. Orthopedics 2008;31:75.
41. Nanavati VN, Werner FW, Sutton LG, et al. Proximal row carpectomy: role of a radiocarpal interposition lateral meniscal allograft. J Hand Surg Am 2009;34:251–7.
42. Kwon BC, Choi SJ, Shin J, et al. Proximal row carpectomy with capsular interposition arthroplasty for advanced arthritis of the wrist. J Bone Joint Surg Br 2009;91:1601–6.
43. Ilyas AM. Proximal row carpectomy with a dorsal capsule interposition flap. Tech Hand Up Extrem Surg 2010;14:136–40.
44. Tang P, Imbriglia JE. Osteochondral resurfacing (OCRPRC) for capitate chondrosis in proximal row carpectomy. J Hand Surg Am 2007;32:1334–42.
45. Eaton RG. Proximal row carpectomy and soft tissue interposition arthroplasty. Tech Hand Up Extrem Surg 1997;1:248–54.

Wrist Arthroplasty
Partial and Total

Brian D. Adams, MD

KEYWORDS

- Wrist arthroplasty • Total wrist arthroplasty • Wrist replacement

KEY POINTS

- Although arthrodesis is the treatment preferred by most surgeons for severe wrist arthritis; some degree of functional impairment occurs from the resulting loss of motion, especially when multiple joints in the extremity are affected by arthritis.
- Total wrist arthroplasty may enhance the performance of daily activities and it is usually preferred by patients over arthrodesis.
- The newer generation of wrist prostheses has demonstrated improved performance and durability in properly selected patients.

INTRODUCTION

The wrist is a common site for arthritis, with 80% of patients with rheumatoid arthritis (RA) complaining of functional impairment caused by wrist pain. Osteoarthritis and posttraumatic arthritis are also common causes for symptomatic wrist pain, particularly in patients with severe scapholunate advanced collapse (SLAC), scaphoid nonunion advanced collapse, and radiocarpal arthritis after severe distal radius fracture. Total wrist arthroplasty has been of interest to clinicians to offer the same benefits provided by arthroplasty of the hip, knee, and shoulder joints. A motion-preserving alternative to wrist arthrodesis is of particular importance when treating patients who are debilitated by arthritis that affects multiple joints. Basic activities of daily living, such as perineal care, fastening buttons, combing hair, and writing, are made easier if some wrist motion is preserved[1,2]; thus, patients with RA typically prefer arthroplasty over arthrodesis to enhance the performance of daily activities.[3–5] Patients with posttraumatic or degenerative osteoarthritis may also select arthroplasty over arthrodesis to better perform specific vocational and avocational activities.

A recent cost-utility analysis[6] compared nonsurgical management, total wrist arthroplasty, and wrist arthrodesis. Hand surgeons, rheumatologists, and patients with RA were given a time trade-off/ utility survey to assess preferences. Results showed that surgical management was preferred to nonsurgical management and was deemed cost-effective by quality-adjusted life-years (QALY). Arthroplasty had a slightly higher cost compared with fusion but not so high as to make it cost prohibitive. Another study by the same group did a utility analysis of rheumatologists and hand surgeons[7] on the treatment of wrist arthritis in patients with RA. The results showed that surgeons and rheumatologists agreed that arthroplasty was the more favorable procedure in expected gain of QALY compared with fusion. Murphy and colleagues[8] compared 24 patients with a wrist arthrodesis and 27 with total wrist arthroplasty and found no difference in overall outcome scores; the arthroplasty patients, however, tended to have greater ease with personal hygiene and selected other tasks and had slightly higher satisfaction overall.

Despite theses potential advantages, wrist arthroplasty has not become a widely accepted

The author receives research funding from Integra Life Sciences, Incorporated, Plainsboro, NJ.
Orthopedic Surgery, University of Iowa, 200 Hawkins Drive Iowa City, IA 52242, USA
E-mail address: brian-d-adams@uiowa.edu

Hand Clin 29 (2013) 79–89
http://dx.doi.org/10.1016/j.hcl.2012.08.029
0749-0712/13/$ – see front matter Published by Elsevier Inc

option by most surgeons, primarily because arthrodesis is simpler to perform and it is more predictable with fewer long-term complications. The natural wrist is a highly complex joint with multiple articulations among of radius, ulna, and carpal bones, which present substantial design challenges in developing implants. Although current arthroplasty designs show improvements over older models, they do not duplicate these interactions. This circumstance results in a variety of compromises in motion, balance, and durability compared with the natural wrist joint. Thus, regardless of the need or desire for arthroplasty, patients must accept and commit to a lifetime of restricted activities imposed by an artificial wrist. Patients must also recognize the risk of implant failure and the possible need for revision surgery.

BRIEF HISTORY

In 1967, Alfred Swanson developed a silicone implant, which became the first widely used implant for wrist arthroplasty.[9] Wrist motion resulted from a combination of implant flexibility and pistoning within the medullary canals of the radius and third metacarpal. These implants often provided initial pain relief and some motion; but restoration of wrist height and hand balance was unpredictable, and follow-up revealed subsidence within the bone and a high incidence of implant breakage, reaching 52% at 72 months.[10–12] Silicone synovitis became an important issue later, although its incidence was lower than with individual carpal bone implants.[13]

The next generation of implants was articulated and used cobalt chrome or titanium and high-density polyethylene. Early articulated designs incorporated bearings with small surface areas to maximize joint motion; however, imbalance and instability were common. A variety of stem designs were developed for cement fixation in the radius and carpus, with carpal components typically fixed in the metacarpal canals. Unfortunately, a high incidence of carpal component loosening occurred, marked by metacarpal erosion, and implant penetration occurred. Periprosthetic bone resorption of the distal radius was also common. An early example was the very popular ball and socket implant introduced by Meuli in 1972.[14] During the same period, Volz developed an articulated unhinged prosthesis with the convex surface on the carpus and the concave surface on the radius. These implants each provided satisfactory early clinical results, but further follow-up revealed continued problems with imbalance, subsidence, and loosening.[15,16] The Biax wrist prosthesis (DePuy, Warsaw, Indiana) had similar fixation but

introduced an ellipsoid-shaped articulation that demonstrated improved wrist balance and the potential for uncemented fixation of the radial component. This implant became very popular, and early results were good in most patients; but loosening remained a substantial problem. Eight out of 11 failures in one series of 58 Biax implants were secondary to distal component loosening and subsidence, which often resulted in penetration through the dorsum of the third metacarpal and substantial bone destruction.[17] The implant has been withdrawn from sale by the manufacturer.

Another attempt to improve on replicating the anatomy is the Anatomic Physiologic implant (Implant-Service Vertreibs-GmbH, Hamburg, Germany) designed with a titanium articulation.[18] Midterm follow-up revealed a very high failure rate, with 39 out of 40 undergoing revision at an average 52-month follow-up. Isolated loosening of the carpal component was the most common mode of failure. Titanium wear debris was found in the soft tissues of all revisions and was thought to be a major contributing factor to early periprosthetic bone resorption.[19]

The Universal wrist (Kinetics Medical, Incorporated, Carlsbad, California) designed by Menon[20] introduced new concepts in total wrist implant design to the United States and is considered the predecessor to current resurfacing-type designs. Although refinements have been made to his design, many of the basic concepts remain, particularly relating to the distal component (**Figs. 1** and **2**).

CURRENT DESIGNS

The overall experience with different designs over the last 3 and a half decades provides evidence that specific criteria must be met to optimize the clinical results. The present generation of prostheses combines many of the basic concepts of the Universal and Biax implants to improve both wrist balance and distal component loosening. Although the natural wrist kinematics are simplified, the designs attempt to replicate the natural center of motion resulting in a functional range of motion and better balance. The articulation is broad, generally ellipsoidal, and semiconstrained to provide a functional range of motion and yet resist imbalance and instability to allow rapid recovery with minimal formal rehabilitation or splint protection.[21]

Distal component fixation is primarily within the carpus and not the metacarpal canals, and screws are used to augment fixation. A key to the durability of distal component fixation is an intercarpal fusion to create a 2-bone wrist joint, eliminating the

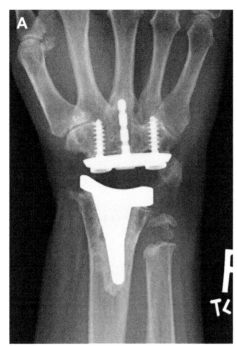
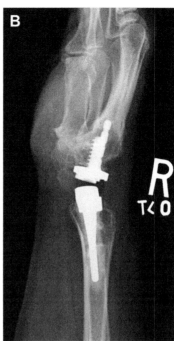

Fig. 1. (*A, B*) Posteroanterior and lateral radiographs of a Kineticos Medical Incorporated total wrist in a 62-year-old woman with inflammatory arthritis at 10-year follow-up. No evidence of loosening or osteolysis.

multiple articulations of the natural wrist. The radial component is shaped to minimize bone resection and preserve the joint capsule to enhance prosthetic stability and wrist balance.

The distal implant component, which must be relatively thin and intricately shaped, is made of titanium for better strength and osteointegration. The proximal component is made of cobalt chrome with a polished articular surface to provide a low friction interface for reduced wear. The articular bearing is made of high-density polyethylene for improved wear characteristics. The articulation is unconstrained, but the concave surface of the radial component provides a stable joint.

Fixation by osteointegration rather than cement is an option for both components in an attempt to improve durability and reduce bone destruction if revision becomes necessary. All systems have the option to preserve the ulnar head and distal radioulnar joint.

There are currently 3 implant systems available in the United States that have used these criteria, but each has unique features. The Remotion total wrist (SBI, New York, New York) offers a mobile bearing attached to the carpal component that theoretically improves motion and load transfer, thus reducing stresses that contribute to loosening.[22] The Universal 2 system (Integra Life Sciences, Plainsboro, New Jersey) is a versatile

system that replicates the natural wrist center of motion and can be used in a wide range of wrists while providing excellent joint stability. The Maestro (Biomet, Warsaw, Indiana) allows complete resection of the proximal carpal row and has a polyethylene surface proximally; it is also approved for hemiarthroplasty using the distal component alone.

PATIENT SELECTION CRITERIA

As with implant arthroplasty of other joints, such as the hip and knee, patient selection is the single most important controllable factor affecting the outcome of total wrist arthroplasty. A variety of patient factors must be included in the decision process but the most important are age; activity demands; bone and soft tissue quality; joint deformity; disease activity; and reliance on the limb for overall body mobility, such as the use of walking aids. In addition, the relative benefits of the procedure compared with other procedures should be considered.

The ideal candidates for a total wrist arthroplasty are patients with a low-demand lifestyle who request relief of pain and are seeking modest wrist motion to retain ease of function for nonstressful activities. Elderly patients with generalized RA have been considered the typical

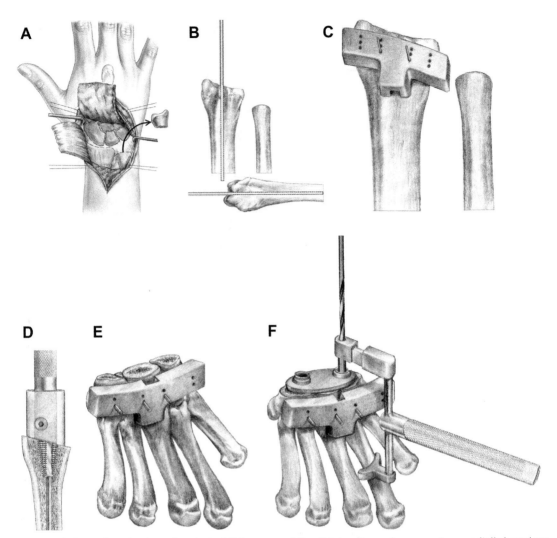

Fig. 2. Technique of total wrist arthroplasty. (*A*) Exposure of the distal radius and carpus using a radially based retinacular flap and distally based capsular flap. Ulnar head excision is optional. (*B*) A guide rod inserted to align cutting block and broach for radius preparation. (*C*) Radial cutting block is applied to resect the articular surface at the proper angle. (*D*) Radius is broached using a cannulated broach over a guide rod. (*E*) A carpal cutting block is applied to guide the osteotomy through the capitate head, scaphoid waist, and midtriquetrum. (*F*) Trial carpal component is inserted and holes are made for the screws using a special drill guide. (*From* Anderson MC, Adams BD. Total wrist arthroplasty. Hand Clin 2005;21(4):621–30; with permission from Elsevier.)

patients indicated for total wrist arthroplasty, particularly those with bilateral wrist arthritis who would otherwise require bilateral wrist fusions. Also, patients with RA with involvement of the hand, elbow, and shoulder often request maintenance of motion in the wrist to better preserve limb function and to avoid a feeling of severe limb stiffness. However, patients with RA with highly active synovitis that is producing bony erosions or joint hyperlaxity have a substantially higher risk of implant instability and loosening and, thus, are better treated by arthrodesis. Regular use of the upper extremities

for support during ambulation or transfers is a contraindication; intermittent use of crutches or a cane, however, is acceptable if patients use a wrist splint.

Patients with posttraumatic or degenerative osteoarthritis may also be candidates for wrist arthroplasty. Because these patients typically have good bone quality, muscle strength, and wrist alignment, the early and midterm results can be excellent. These patients, however, should choose arthroplasty to maintain dexterity for activities of daily living and specific low-demand activities rather than to increase activity levels and perform stressful tasks with less pain. Patients with osteoarthritis who have highly demanding lifestyles are not good candidates. Many patients with posttraumatic arthritis are young and very active and, thus, are not candidates for arthroplasty because of the high stresses they will likely impose on the wrist.

Absolute contraindications for total wrist arthroplasty include a minimally functional hand, recent infection, and lack of wrist extension power caused by ruptures of the extensor carpi radialis brevis and longus tendons or radial nerve palsy.

Patients should undergo a routine preoperative evaluation. In patients with RA, the cervical spine is evaluated for instability with flexion and extension views to ensure their safety under anesthesia. Physical examination of the wrist confirms active wrist extensor power and functional digits. Failure to recognize preoperative soft tissue contractures may lead to persistent wrist deformity, reduced wrist motion, and imbalance of the extrinsic finger tendons. Posteroanterior and lateral views of the wrist are reviewed to assess bone stock, joint deformity, and probable implant size. There must be adequate bone stock and quality to support the implant, especially the distal component. Implantation in patients with severe osteopenia, bone erosion, or joint deformity is more challenging; and the implant fixation is likely less durable. Previous surgical fusion or proximal row carpectomy are relative contraindications; these patients must have adequate carpus remaining and intact wrist extensors.

Lower limb surgery, such as total hip or knee arthroplasty, should be done before wrist replacement to avoid weight bearing on the wrist replacement during rehabilitation of the lower limb. Procedures on the digits should be completed after wrist arthroplasty to optimize joint alignment and tendon balance in the hand.

If bone loss or active erosive disease of the carpus is suspected but not confirmed by preoperative imaging, a complete arthrodesis is discussed with patients preoperatively as an alternative procedure that will be based on an intraoperative assessment. Partial or complete resection of the distal ulna is planned when there is symptomatic arthritis of the distal radioulnar joint, but otherwise the wrist arthroplasty technique should avoid violating the distal radioulnar joint. The implant size is estimated using radiographic templates, but the final size is often determined during surgery.

SURGICAL TECHNIQUE
Step 1: Setup and Incision

Although the technique for the Universal 2 is described, the basic principles apply to other wrist

arthroplasty systems. Prophylactic antibiotics are administered. The operation is performed under general or axillary regional anesthesia, and a nonsterile arm tourniquet is used. A strip of transparent adhesive film is applied to the dorsum of the hand and wrist to protect the skin from damage during instrumentation.

A dorsal longitudinal incision is made over the wrist in line with the third metacarpal. The skin and subcutaneous tissue are elevated from the extensor retinaculum and held with retraction sutures. Care is taken to protect branches of the superficial radial nerve and dorsal cutaneous branches of the ulnar nerve. If the distal ulna is to be resected, the extensor carpi ulnaris compartment is opened along its volar margin. Alternatively, if the distal radioulnar joint is to be preserved, the extensor digitorum quinti is opened dorsally. The extensor retinaculum is elevated radially to the septum between the first and second extensor compartments. An extensor tenosynovectomy is performed if needed and the tendons are retracted.

Step 2: Joint Exposure

A distally based rectangular flap of joint capsule is raised over the dorsal wrist. The sides of the flap are made along the far medial and lateral aspects of the wrist. If the ulnar head is to be resected, the proximal edge of the capsule is raised in continuity with the dorsal capsule of the distal radioulnar joint and the periosteum over the distal 1 cm of the distal radius to create a long and broad flap for closure over the prosthesis. If the distal ulna is to be preserved, then the interval between the capsule and the dorsal distal radioulnar ligament is carefully divided and the capsule is raised distally to preserve the horizontal components of the triangular fibrocartilage complex. The brachioradialis and the tendons of the first dorsal compartment are elevated subperiosteally from the distal part of the radial styloid. The wrist is fully flexed to expose the joint. Synovectomies of the radiocarpal and distal radioulnar joints are performed when needed. A partial or complete distal ulna resection is performed if needed at this time.

Step 3: Preparation of the Radius

Using a bone awl or drill, a hole is made through the articular surface of the radius about 5 mm below its dorsal rim and under the Lister tubercle. The hole is enlarged and the radial alignment guide advanced into the medullary canal. Fluoroscopy is used to confirm that the guide rod is centered within the canal. The cutting guides are applied and aligned to resect a minimum amount of distal radius to create a flat distal surface. The radius cut is completed, but the sigmoid notch is preserved by stopping the cut a few millimeters short of the distal radioulnar joint. The radial component is designed with an ulnar-sided flare to avoid the distal radioulnar joint. The alignment rod is reinserted and the proper-sized broach head is used. Its orientation is important to reproduce the natural, slightly supinated position of the carpus relative to the radius. A trial radial component is inserted. The carpus can be reduced on the radial component to assess soft tissue tension. If it is excessive, then further resection of the radius may be necessary but is usually delayed until the carpal preparation is completed.

Step 4: Preparation of the Carpus

If the scaphoid and triquetrum are mobile, carpus preparation is facilitated by first temporarily pinning these bones to the capitate and hamate. The lunate is excised by sharp dissection. Using the drill guide, a guide wire is inserted in the capitate along the long axis of the third metacarpal. Fluoroscopy is used to confirm the proper position of the wire. A cannulated drill is used to create a hole. The cutting guides are applied and aligned to make the cut through the proximal 1 mm of the hamate, a small amount of the capitate head, and about half of the scaphoid and triquetrum. The trial component is inserted. Screw holes for the carpal component can be made at this time or at the time of final implant insertion depending on surgeon preference. The holes are typically not perpendicular to the carpal component, with the radial screw extending into the base of the second metacarpal and the ulnar screw passing into the body of the hamate but not into the fourth metacarpal.

Step 5: Trial Reduction

A trial polyethylene is applied to the carpal plate, and the range of motion and stability are checked. The prosthesis should demonstrate approximately 35° of flexion and extension with modest tightness at full extension. If the volar capsule is limiting extension, then the radius may be shortened slightly but no more than 2 mm at a time. When a preoperative flexion contracture is present, a step-cut tendon lengthening of the wrist flexors may be necessary. Conversely, when tension is insufficient, the palmar joint capsule is inspected and repaired when detached. If the capsule is intact but instability persists, then a thicker polyethylene component may be required.

Step 6: Implantation

Before implantation, 3 horizontal mattress sutures of 2-0 polyester are placed through small bone holes along the dorsal rim of the distal radius for later capsule closure. If the ulnar head was resected, then sutures are also placed through the dorsal part of the ulna neck. The dorsal portions of the articular surfaces are removed from the triquetrum, capitate, hamate, scaphoid, and trapezoid; and previously resected bone is packed into the spaces to achieve an intercarpal arthrodesis. The final implants are impacted into place, and the final screws are inserted. The appropriate polyethylene component is applied to the carpal plate, and a final assessment of motion and stability is made.

Step 7: Closure

If the distal ulna was resected, the palmar capsule on the ulnar aspect of the wrist is brought dorsally and sutured to the end of the ulna through drill holes. The dorsal wrist capsule is reattached to the distal margin of the radius and ulna using the previously placed sutures. If the capsule is deficient, the extensor retinaculum is divided in line with its fibers and one-half is placed under the tendons to cover the prosthesis. Meticulous closure of the capsule is mandatory to ensure prosthetic stability and to protect the tendons from irritation. The remaining retinaculum is repaired, leaving the extensor carpi radialis longus and brevis and the extensor pollicis longus superficial to the retinaculum. The skin is closed over a self-suction drain, and the wrist is immobilized in a bulky gauze dressing and a plaster splint. Because the procedure may be associated with substantial postoperative swelling, strict elevation of the hand and immediate active finger motion are very important.

POSTOPERATIVE MANAGEMENT AND REHABILITATION

The dressing and plaster splint are removed between 2 and 10 days after the procedure, and a removable well-molded wrist splint is applied. A supervised exercise program is initiated consisting of full digital motion and gentle active wrist and forearm motion that emphasizes wrist extension but avoids forceful wrist flexion until 4 weeks after the procedure to protect the capsule repair. Patients are gradually weaned from the splint after 4 weeks, and strengthening is added. Full activities are permitted after 8 weeks depending on discomfort and swelling. Patients are advised to avoid impact loading of the wrist (eg, use of a hammer, playing tennis) and repetitive forceful use of the hand.

Permanent restrictions are lifting limited to 10 lb on an occasional basis and 2 lb on a regular basis.

OUTCOMES

There have been relatively few published reports on the outcomes of presently available prostheses, but several studies have been published on the outcomes of the Universal wrist designed by Menon. In Menon's first report of 37 Universal prostheses with a mean follow-up of 6.7 years (range 4–10 years), none of the cases demonstrated radiographic evidence of distal component loosening.[20] A further follow-up study that included 57 implants again demonstrated no evidence of carpal component loosening.[23] Subsidence of the radial component was observed but was not progressive or symptomatic. Consistently good pain relief (90%) and a functional range of motion was achieved, with an average postoperative motion of 36° extension, 41° flexion, 7° radial deviation, and 13° ulnar deviation. Dislocation was the most common complication, with 5 occurring in the first 37 cases and a total of 6 among the 57 cases in the later follow-up. The initial higher incidence of dislocation was partly attributed to the lack of availability of different implant sizes and thicknesses of polyethylene inserts at that time.

A prospective study of 22 Universal prosthesis implanted by 2 surgeons with a 1- to 2-year follow-up demonstrated results similar to Menon's. Patients achieved an average of 41° flexion and 35° extension.[24] Disabilities of the Arm, Shoulder, and Hand (DASH) outcome survey scores improved 24 points at 2 years. Three prostheses (14%) were unstable and required further treatment; all 3 were in patients with highly active rheumatoid disease with severe wrist laxity.[22]

Ward and colleagues[25,26] reported a prospective consecutive series of 25 wrist arthroplasties in 21 patients with RA. Fifteen patients (19 wrists) returned for clinical and radiographic examination at a mean of follow-up of 7.6 years (range 5.0–10.8 years). Mean wrist flexion and extension at the final follow-up were 42° and 20°, respectively, for a mean improvement in the total flexion-extension arc of 14°. The average DASH score improved from 62 points preoperatively to 40 points at 5 years after surgery. A total of 9 wrists in 8 patients had undergone revision surgery for a loose carpal component. Two additional wrists in 2 patients had radiographic evidence of carpal component subsidence at the final follow-up. The investigators concluded that the Universal wrist prosthesis provided a functional range of motion and good patient-reported outcome measures in patients with a functioning implant. Carpal

component loosening led to a high incidence of failure, resulting in revision surgery in 47% of the patients by 10 years. However, most failures occurred in patients with severe and persistently active rheumatoid disease who would, by today's criteria, no longer be considered candidates for wrist arthroplasty, whereas those with less severe and better controlled disease had durable outcomes.

The author's early results were reviewed for the Universal 2 prosthesis (**Fig. 3**) in 25 wrists: 20 patients had RA, 2 had posttraumatic arthritis, and 3 had osteoarthritis.[27] Twenty patients were women and 5 were men. All prostheses were implanted uncemented. Results showed functional motion, with an average of 37° flexion, 33° extension, 22° ulnar deviation, and 9° radial deviation. Motion often did not maximize for 6 months. Pain relief was rated good by all patients, but mild ulnar-sided wrist discomfort persisted in 5 patients. The average DASH score improved 20% and the Patient-Rated Wrist Evaluation score improved 35%. No patients showed radiographic implant loosening, but 3 patients with osteopenia had 2 to 5 mm of subsidence, which plateaued after 1 year. The carpal component stem fractured in 3 patients who had the first version of this implant. All were revised and recovered a functional result. Very soon after the initial release, the implant was subsequently redesigned with a greater diameter (stronger) stem and full porous coating over the distal surface (stem and plate) to better share and transfer the load to the carpus. No fractures have been found with the new version of the carpal component.

Ferreres and colleagues[28] published a review of 21 consecutive Universal 2 implants with an average 5.5-year follow-up. Most of the patients had inflammatory arthritis, but 4 patients had chondrocalcinosis, grade IV Kienboeck disease, or degenerative arthritis. Only 1 patient reported not being satisfied with the procedure, and 11 reported being very satisfied. Average flexion and extension range of motion was reported as 42° and 26°, respectively. No patient had a dislocation or revision surgery in the follow-up period, but 2 had radiographic osteolysis and 1 had subsidence of the distal component.

Herzberg[22] reported the early results using the Remotion prostheses. The series included 20 wrists of which 13 were in patients with RA. The patients were prospectively followed for a minimum of 12 months, with an average of 32 months. There was one carpal and one radial component loosening, both in patients with RA. Patients with RA had an average 41% improvement in clinical scores, with 7 excellent, 5 good,

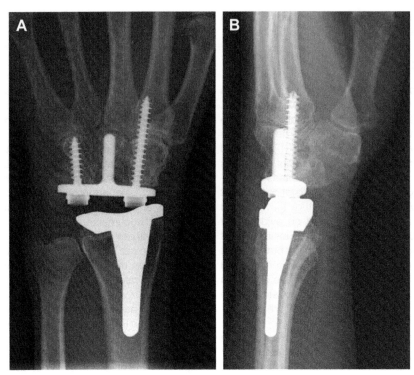

Fig. 3. (A, B) Posteroanterior and lateral radiographs of a Universal 2 total wrist in a 59-year-old woman with RA at 7-year follow-up. No evidence of loosening or osteolysis.

and 1 poor result. The patients without RA had an average 27% improvement in clinical scores, with 2 excellent, 2 good, 2 fair, and 1 poor result. Overall, there was significant improvement in pain and function but only modest improvement in strength. The investigators concluded that the Remotion wrist showed better outcomes than older designs and similar to the Universal 2.

PARTIAL WRIST ARTHROPLASTY (HEMIARTHROPLASTY)

Although total wrist arthroplasty has been used in selected patients with advanced arthritis, high-demand patients are infrequently considered primarily because of a high risk for implant loosening, particularly of the distal component. A distal radius hemiarthroplasty may obviate the strict restrictions required of patients treated by total wrist arthroplasty. It may provide another motion-preserving surgical option for active patients with severe wrist arthritis, especially those with distal radius articular degeneration from osteoarthritis or those with posttraumatic arthritis.

Using this concept, the author has performed a combined proximal row carpectomy and hemiarthroplasty using the radial component of the Universal 2 wrist.[29] The first patient was a 42-year-old woman with RA and bilateral severe

wrist arthritis showing distal radius erosion and volar carpal subluxation but good condition of the capitate on the first side (**Fig. 4**). She obtained good pain relief and an 80° flexion-extension arc at a 2-year follow-up. The second patient was a man with an SLAC wrist who, at the 1-year follow-up, denied pain and had a 69° flexion-extension arc. The procedure has subsequently been done in 26 wrists in 24 patients, with up to a 3-year follow-up. Initial selection criteria for the first 5 patients included a capitate head having only minimal articular cartilage changes, but this was subsequently changed to a capitate without erosion or cystic changes. The diagnoses were RA in 2 patients (3 wrists), SLAC wrist in 18 (19 wrists), and posttraumatic in 4 patients (4 wrists). The procedure generated a minimum of 30° each of flexion and extension in 22 out of the 26 wrists. The patients that failed to achieve this range of motion were 2 patients with RA, 1 with an SLAC wrist, and 1 with posttraumatic arthritis. The patient with RA ultimately underwent a revision to a complete arthrodesis because of continued synovitis and erosions throughout the carpus. The patient with the SLAC wrist had preoperative cystic changes in the capitate and is showing erosion of the capitate at the 1-year follow-up but remains satisfied with the procedure at this time. The other 2 patients remain satisfied with

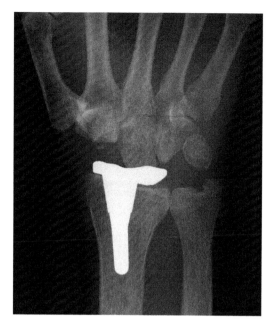

Fig. 4. Hemiarthroplasty using the radius component only of a Universal total wrist combined with a proximal row carpectomy in a 65-year-old man at 3-year follow-up.

their outcomes, including good pain relief despite reduced motion. In retrospect, the 2 wrists showing postoperative changes of the capitate also had poor structural bone quality preoperatively and should not have been indicated for the procedure. However, both patients had a satisfactory result on the first wrist and requested the procedure on the opposite side. The remaining patients are showing no measureable capitate erosion or loss of motion.

COMPLICATIONS AND MANAGEMENT OF FAILED WRIST ARTHROPLASTY

A comprehensive review of strategies for the prevention and management of intraoperative and postoperative complications in total wrist arthroplasty is beyond the scope of this article but can be found in other reports.[30,31] Potential intraoperative complications include fractures and tendon injury. Early postoperative complications include wound-healing problems (hematoma, wound edge necrosis, dehiscence), extensor tendon adhesions, wrist stiffness, wrist imbalance, distal radioulnar joint problems (impingement, instability, arthrosis), prosthetic instability, and infection. The most common long-term serious complication is implant loosening, particularly of the distal component in the newer designs. Osteolysis can occur because of polyethylene wear, with

concurrent metallosis if the polyethylene wear results in exposed metal surfaces (**Fig. 5**). Metallosis can also occur from screw carpal plate interface motion caused by carpal component loosening. The true incidence of these complications for the newest designs of wrist replacement remains unknown in the absence of adequate long-term reports.

Revision arthroplasty, arthrodesis, and resection arthroplasty are options for salvaging a failed total wrist arthroplasty caused by imbalance, loosening, or instability.[30,31] Revision arthroplasty is an option for aseptic loosening if there is adequate bone stock or if bone grafting is feasible. The thickened capsule must be widely released to allow wrist flexion and extraction of the components. If there has been substantial subsidence, then lengthening of the wrist flexors and extensor tendons may be required. Iliac crest bone graft may be needed to fill defects and reestablish the basic architecture of the carpus. When using the Universal 2 prosthesis for revision, the graft can be transfixed to the remaining carpus using the carpal component fixation screws. Because the decision to perform a revision depends primarily on the integrity of the bone and soft tissues, it may not be possible to decide until direct inspection at the time of surgery. Thus, the surgeon must

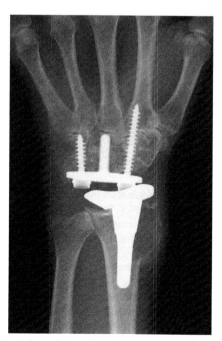

Fig. 5. Universal 2 total wrist in a 63-year-old woman with RA at 7-year follow-up showing severe osteolysis. Carpal component remained well fixed. Joint was debrided and defects filled with allograft. Polyethylene bearing component was revised.

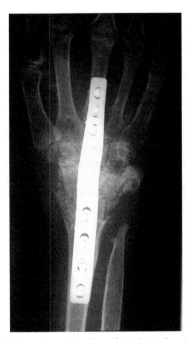

Fig. 6. Wrist arthrodesis for a failed total wrist using the cancellous portion only of a femoral head allograft and a dorsal wrist arthrodesis plate.

be prepared for arthroplasty and for arthrodesis. Patients who have poor bone stock, severe capsule defects, or particulate synovitis are rarely indicated for revision arthroplasty. Removal of the implant components, intercalary bone graft using the cancellous portion only of a femoral head allograft shaped to fill the defect, and dorsal arthrodesis plate is an effective technique though the time to fusion can be several months (**Fig. 6**). An established infection should be treated by implant removal and primary or delayed conversion to an arthrodesis.

SUMMARY

Total wrist arthroplasty preserves motion and improves hand function for daily tasks and lower-demand vocational and avocational activities. It is often preferable to fusion when both wrists are arthritic. Early implant designs were troubled by complications, including wrist imbalance and loosening; however, newer prosthetic designs provide a functional range of motion, better wrist balance, reduced risk of loosening, and better implant stability. The procedure is more likely to be successful in lower-demand patients. Complications are less common in patients with adequate bone stock and who do not have severe wrist deformity or highly active disease. In properly selected patients, short-term complications are uncommon.

The success of total wrist arthroplasty depends on appropriate patient selection, careful preoperative planning, and sound surgical technique.

REFERENCES

1. Murray PM. Current status of wrist arthrodesis and wrist arthroplasty. Clin Plast Surg 1996;23:385–94.
2. Goodman M, Millender LH, Nalebuff ED, et al. Arthroplasty of the rheumatoid wrist with silicone rubber: an early evaluation. J Hand Surg Am 1980; 5(2):114–21.
3. Vicar AJ, Burton RI. Surgical management of rheumatoid wrist fusion or arthroplasty. J Hand Surg Am 1986;11:790–7.
4. Kobus RI, Turner RH. Wrist arthrodesis for treatment of rheumatoid arthritis. J Hand Surg Am 1990;15: 541–6.
5. Weiss AC, Wiedeman GJ, Quenzer D, et al. Upper extremity function after wrist arthrodesis. J Hand Surg Am 1995;20:813–7.
6. Cavaliere CM, Chung KC. A cost-utility analysis of nonsurgical management, total wrist arthroplasty, and total wrist arthrodesis in rheumatoid arthritis. J Hand Surg Am 2010;35:379–91.
7. Cavaliere CM, Oppenheimer AJ, Chung KC. Reconstructing the rheumatoid wrist: a utility analysis comparing total wrist fusion and total wrist arthroplasty from the perspectives of rheumatologists and hand surgeons. Hand (N Y) 2010;5:9–18.
8. Murphy DM, Khoury JG, Imbriglia JE, et al. Comparison of arthroplasty and arthrodesis in rheumatoid arthritis. J Hand Surg Am 2003;28:570–6.
9. Swanson AB. Flexible implant arthroplasty for arthritic disabilities of the radiocarpal joint. A silicone rubber intramedullary stemmed flexible hinge implant for the wrist joint. Orthop Clin North Am 1973;4(2):383–94.
10. Jolly SL, Ferlic DC, Calyton ML, et al. Swanson silicone arthroplasty of the wrist in rheumatoid arthritis: a long-term follow-up. J Hand Surg Am 1992;17(1): 142–9.
11. Fatti JF, Palmer AK, Mosher JF. The long-term results of Swanson silicone rubber interpositional wrist arthroplasty. J Hand Surg Am 1986;11(2):166–75.
12. Stanley JK, Tolat AR. Long-term results of Swanson silastic arthroplasty in the rheumatoid wrist. J Hand Surg Br 1993;18(3):381–8.
13. Peimer CA, Medige J, Eckert BS, et al. Reactive synovitis after silicone arthroplasty. J Hand Surg Am 1986;11(5):624–38.
14. Meuli HC. Total wrist arthroplasty. Experience with a noncemented wrist prosthesis. Clin Orthop 1997; 342:77–83.
15. Dennis DA, Ferlic DC, Clayton ML. Volz total wrist arthroplasty in rheumatoid arthritis: a long-term review. J Hand Surg Am 1986;11:483–9.

16. Menon J. Total wrist replacement using the modified Volz prosthesis. J Bone Joint Surg Am 1987; 69:998–1006.
17. Cobb TK, Beckenbaugh RD. Biaxial total-wrist arthroplasty. J Hand Surg Am 1996;21(6):1011–21.
18. Radmer S, Andresen R, Sparmann M. Wrist arthroplasty with a new generation of prostheses in patients with rheumatoid arthritis. J Hand Surg Am 1999;24(5):935–43.
19. Radmer S, Andresen R, Sparmann M. Total wrist arthroplasty in patients with rheumatoid arthritis. J Hand Surg Am 2003;28(5):789–94.
20. Menon J. Universal total wrist implant. Experience with a carpal component fixed with three screws. J Arthroplasty 1998;13:515–23.
21. Grosland NM, Rogge RD, Adams BD. Influence of articular geometry on prosthetic wrist stability. Clin Orthop 2004;421:134–42.
22. Herzberg G. Prospective study of a new total wrist arthroplasty: short-term results. Chir Main 2011; 30(1):20–5.
23. Menon J. Total wrist arthroplasty for rheumatoid arthritis. In: Saffar P, Foucher G, Amadio PC, editors. Current Practice in Hand Surgery. Martin Dunitz: London; 1997. p. 209–14.
24. Divelbiss BJ, Sollerman C, Adams BD. Early results of the Universal total wrist arthroplasty in rheumatoid arthritis. J Hand Surg Am 2002;27:195–204.
25. Ward CM, Kuhl TL, Adams BD. Five to ten-year outcomes of the Universal total wrist arthroplasty in patients with rheumatoid arthritis. J Bone Joint Surg Am 2011;93:914–9.
26. Conaway DA, Kuhl TL, Adams BD. Comparison of the native ulnar head and a partial ulnar head resurfacing implant. J Hand Surg Am 2009;34(6): 1056–62.
27. Anderson MC, Adams BD. Total wrist arthroplasty. Hand Clin 2005;21(4):621–30.
28. Ferreres A, Lluch A, del Valle M. Universal total wrist arthroplasty: midterm follow-up study. J Hand Surg Am 2011;36:967–73.
29. Boyer JS, Adams BD. Distal radius hemiarthroplasty combined with proximal row carpectomy: case report. Iowa Orthop J 2010;30:168–73.
30. Adams BD. Complications of wrist arthroplasty. Hand Clin 2010;26:213–20.
31. Rizzo M, Ackerman DB, Rodrigues RL, et al. Wrist arthrodesis as a salvage procedure for failed implant arthroplasty. J Hand Surg Eur Vol 2011; 36(1):29–33.

Prosthetic Arthroplasty of the Distal Radioulnar Joint
Historical Perspective and 24-Year Follow-Up

Marwan A. Wehbé, MD[a,b],*

KEYWORDS

- Arthroplasty • Ulna • Ulnar head • Sigmoid notch • Joint replacement • Radioulnar joint
- Distal radioulnar joint • DRUJ

KEY POINTS

- This is a report of the first prosthetic hemiarthroplasty and full arthroplasty, designed and implanted for the distal radioulnar joint in 1988.
- Two case reports are presented, with follow-up of 24 years.
- Experience and problems in the design of both a hemiarthroplasty and total prosthetic arthroplasty are described, in the hope that future developments may avoid past failures.

There has recently been a flurry of activity directed at prosthetic replacement of the distal radioulnar joint (DRUJ). A variety of designs have been marketed after a short period of trial and short follow-up of patients. Lessons from past failures may help avoid failures in future designs.

The DRUJ is an important element of forearm rotation. Salvage procedures for the DRUJ fall into 2 categories: fusion or resection arthroplasty. Fusion of that joint can be disabling because of the loss of forearm rotation, so a great deal of effort has been spent developing various arthroplasties. The ulnar head resection has been the standard for arthroplasty, and numerous variations of that procedure have been described.[1,2] Since the failed silicone arthroplasty was abandoned, few reports could be found until recently describing attempts at prosthetic replacement. This article describes the early development and long-term result of prosthetic arthroplasty.

CASE 1

A 25-year-old right-handed black male machine operator sustained blunt trauma to his left wrist in 1984. When he was first seen, 2 years after the injury, he had already undergone a silicone resection arthroplasty of the DRUJ but continued to complain of clicking and pain in his wrist, primarily with forearm rotation (**Fig. 1**). Two attempts at stabilizing his distal ulna failed to alleviate his pain, so he underwent a prosthetic hemiarthroplasty in February, 1988 (**Fig. 2**).

After surgery, he was immobilized in a plaster sugar-tong splint for 1 month, after which he achieved full range of motion (**Fig. 3**). He continued to have occasional clicking and pain with forearm rotation. Four years later, a total joint replacement was designed for him, but could not be inserted because the original implant was solidly incorporated into the ulna shaft, so the DRUJ joint was debrided. The clicking and the pain improved, and he was happy living in that condition until he fell on that wrist another 4 years later. Radiographs obtained at that time revealed a lytic lesion at the distal end of the resected ulna. This lesion was treated expectantly, but seemed to get larger over a 2-year period (**Fig. 4**). The lesion was excised and packed with olecranon bone graft. It contained synovial-like fluid; cultures were negative.

Disclaimer: Author has no financial interests to disclose.
[a] Pennsylvania Hand Center, 101 South Bryn Mawr Avenue, Suite 300, Bryn Mawr, PA 19010, USA; [b] Jefferson Medical College, Philadelphia, PA, USA
* Pennsylvania Hand Center, 101 South Bryn Mawr Avenue, Suite 300, Bryn Mawr, PA 19010.
E-mail address: marwan.wehbe@pahandcenter.com

Hand Clin 29 (2013) 91–101
http://dx.doi.org/10.1016/j.hcl.2012.08.024
0749-0712/13/$ – see front matter © 2013 Elsevier Inc. All rights reserved.

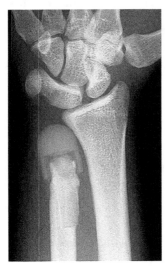

Fig. 1. Case 1: 12 months after silicone ulnar head arthroplasty and persistent gross instability. (*Courtesy of* Pennsylvania Hand Center, Bryn Mawr, PA, USA; with permission.)

In August, 2002, this patient had pain with extremes of forearm rotation, and was considering a revision of the arthroplasty or radioulnar fusion. The implant was removed on October 2, 2003 (15 years after implantation) (**Fig. 5**). The bony ingrowth around the prosthesis stem prevented its complete removal, and a decision was made to cut that stem, keep it in place, and incorporate it in the new prosthesis design. A new total DRUJ prosthesis was designed for him and implanted on October 4, 2004 (**Fig. 6**). Postoperatively, he was immobilized with a sugar-tong plaster splint for 3.5 weeks, after which protected range of motion was started. By 8 weeks after surgery, he developed massive swelling in his hand and wrist, which could not be controlled by nonoperative means (**Fig. 7**). An open debridement was performed at 4 months and again at

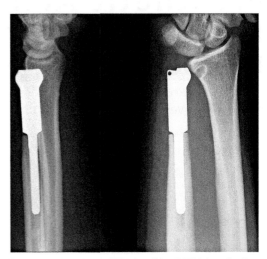

Fig. 2. Case 1: immediately after DRUJ hemiarthroplasty (1988). (*Courtesy of* Pennsylvania Hand Center, Bryn Mawr, PA, USA; with permission.)

10 months. Massive metallic staining was found throughout the operative field, and the swelling persisted. Metal allergy was suspected, even though skin testing was negative. The prosthesis was removed 1 year after implantation, and all swelling promptly resolved (**Fig. 8**). His range of motion returned to normal, and his DRUJ instability and pain recurred. On March 12, 2008, he underwent a Scheker total DRUJ arthroplasty, and maintained a full range of motion with no pain, 18 months later (**Fig. 9**).

CASE 2

This right-handed white female nurse was 51 years old in February, 1991, when she underwent a prosthetic ulna hemiarthroplasty. She had sustained a left wrist fracture at age 15 years, had her ulnar head excised at age 18 years, and a fibula graft at age 26 years, in an attempt to stabilize her

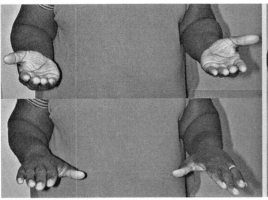
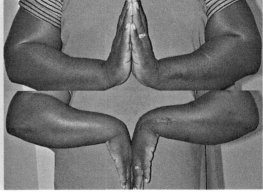

Fig. 3. Case 1: range of motion 5 months after hemiarthroplasty. This degree of motion has persisted until the present time. (*Courtesy of* Pennsylvania Hand Center, Bryn Mawr, PA, USA; with permission.)

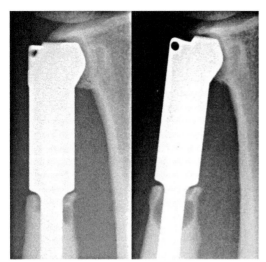

Fig. 4. Case 1: 8 years after hemiarthroplasty, a lytic lesion is evident in the distal ulna. The lesion was larger 2 years later. (*Courtesy of* Pennsylvania Hand Center, Bryn Mawr, PA, USA; with permission.)

DRUJ. The graft was removed 6 years later, and she underwent a left wrist fusion along with a silicone ulna head arthroplasty at age 36 years. When first seen at age 48 years, she had gross instability of the DRUJ with pain (**Fig. 10**).

In the course of the prosthetic arthroplasty, the medullary canal was found to be occluded because of her multiple previous surgeries, and a cortical fracture was produced when the distal ulna was reamed with flexible reamers (**Fig. 11**). Nevertheless, the procedure was completed, and the patient was immobilized with a plaster sugar-tong splint for 4 months, after which protected

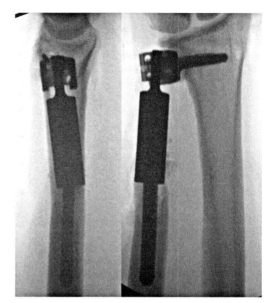

Fig. 6. Case 1: radiographs obtained after total DRUJ arthroplasty. (*Courtesy of* Pennsylvania Hand Center, Bryn Mawr, PA, USA; with permission.)

range of motion was started. At 11 months postoperatively, she had full pronation and 45° of supination (**Fig. 12**).

This patient returned 10 years postoperatively with a ganglion cyst in the opposite wrist (right). Radiographs of the left wrist obtained at that time (10 years after arthroplasty) revealed loosening of the implant, with windshield wiper effect (**Fig. 13**). Twenty-one years after DRUJ arthroplasty, she was totally asymptomatic and still had full forearm rotation on that side with no instability, and she declined any treatment (**Fig. 14**).

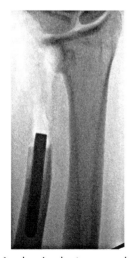

Fig. 5. Case 1: ulna implant removed, but with retained stem. (*Courtesy of* Pennsylvania Hand Center, Bryn Mawr, PA, USA; with permission.)

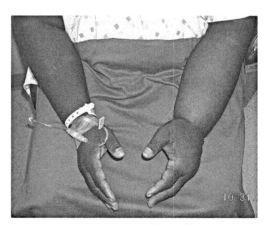

Fig. 7. Case 1: prominent swelling of hand and forearm, which persisted for 1 year, despite hand therapy, medication, and surgical debridements. (*Courtesy of* Pennsylvania Hand Center, Bryn Mawr, PA, USA; with permission.)

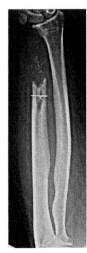

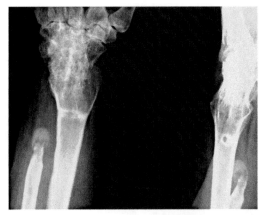

Fig. 10. Case 2: 12 years after ulnar head silicone arthroplasty and gross instability. (*Courtesy of* Pennsylvania Hand Center, Bryn Mawr, PA, USA; with permission.)

tool, to be used in conjunction with a sliding hammer (**Fig. 16**).

Fig. 8. Case 1: all metal has been removed. Some metal staining of the soft tissues remains. Intraoperative fracture of the distal ulna was fixed with a circlage wire. (*Courtesy of* Pennsylvania Hand Center, Bryn Mawr, PA, USA; with permission.)

THE PROSTHESIS
Hemiarthroplasty

The implant for both of these cases was custom-made in 1988 (Biomet, Warsaw, IN) based on measurements taken from the normal contralateral wrist. The prosthesis was made with a titanium alloy, with porous plasma spray stem to allow bony ingrowth. An eyelet was created on the ulnar head for ligament anchor and for implant extraction (**Fig. 15**).

An indentation in the distal end of the implant allowed for impaction of the implant, with a custom

Total Joint Replacement: Sigmoid Notch

A 2-part implant was designed in 1992 for use in the proposed revision of case 1. The ulnar component was identical to the hemiarthroplasty (**Fig. 17**). The radial (sigmoid notch) component consisted of a metallic plate with a polyethylene insert. The plate was titanium-based, with a plasma-sprayed central peg and 2 screw holes. Two different thickness polyethylene inserts were designed to snap into the central peg, to accommodate the spacing between the ulnar head and sigmoid notch. This component was designed for insertion before the final seating of the ulna prosthesis. That implant was never used, because

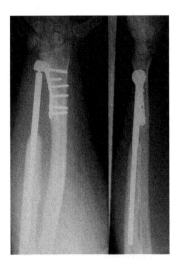

Fig. 9. Case 1: Aptis prosthesis (Aptis Medical, Glenview, KY) helped resolve pain and instability and maintained full range of motion. (*Courtesy of* Pennsylvania Hand Center, Bryn Mawr, PA, USA; with permission.)

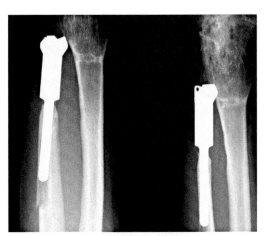

Fig. 11. Case 2: immediately after DRUJ hemiarthroplasty (1991). Distal ulna fracture is obvious. (*Courtesy of* Pennsylvania Hand Center, Bryn Mawr, PA, USA; with permission.)

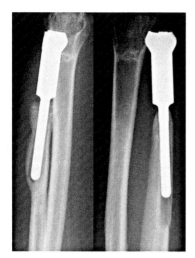

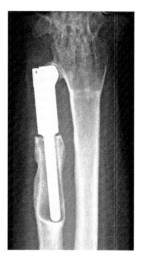

Fig. 12. Case 2: distal ulna fracture healed uneventfully; range of motion was started 5 months postoperatively and reached 80° of pronation and 45° of supination 11 months after surgery. (*Courtesy of* Pennsylvania Hand Center, Bryn Mawr, PA, USA; with permission.)

Fig. 13. Case 2: 11 years after arthroplasty, windshield wiper appearance of lytic lesion in the distal ulna indicates gross motion of the implant, and absence of bony ingrowth. (*Courtesy of* Pennsylvania Hand Center, Bryn Mawr, PA, USA; with permission.)

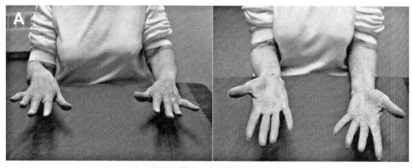

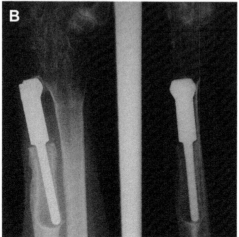

Fig. 14. Case 2: (*A*) the patient returned because of contralateral wrist pain. Full forearm rotation was maintained until the present time. Wrist range of motion is limited by the old fusion. (*B*) Radiograph 21 years after surgery shows no change in distal ulna, when compared with 10 years earlier.

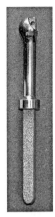

Fig. 15. Mark 1 prosthesis for DRUJ hemiarthroplasty (1988). The stem has plasma spray for bony ingrowth and an eyelet, which may be used for extraction. (*Courtesy of* Pennsylvania Hand Center, Bryn Mawr, PA, USA; with permission.)

the ulnar component could not be removed at surgery.

A second design was made, for a semiconstrained total joint replacement (**Fig. 18**). That implant included a polyethylene bushing, as interface between the 2 metallic components. The implant was used on only 1 occasion, and had to be removed because of metal synovitis, as described in case 1.

DISCUSSION

The DRUJ is a major element of forearm rotation. Its integrity depends on a bowed radius, which rotates around a relatively stable and immobile ulna. Distally, the ulnar head articulates with the sigmoid notch of

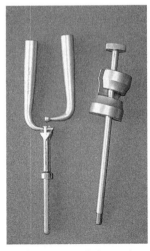

Fig. 16. Sliding hammer with impaction and extraction tool attachments. (*Courtesy of* Pennsylvania Hand Center, Bryn Mawr, PA, USA; with permission.)

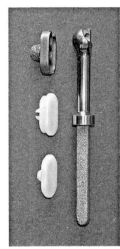

Fig. 17. Mark 2 total DRUJ arthroplasty (1992) added a radius sigmoid notch component, consisting of a metallic plate and different thickness polyethylene inserts. (*Courtesy of* Pennsylvania Hand Center, Bryn Mawr, PA, USA; with permission.)

the radius. The stability of that joint is the result of forearm connections: interosseous membrane, pronator quadratus muscle, and extensor carpi ulnaris (ECU) tendon and various components of the triangular fibrocartilage (TFC) complex.

DRUJ disorders can be the result of bone length discrepancy (ulna variance) or shape disorder (loss of radial bow or ulnar linearity). This situation results in loss of forearm rotation or wrist motion, and possibly pain. Joint factors, such as incongruity (eg, after fracture) or chondromalacia (as after trauma, inflammation, or infection) are likely to cause pain, with minimal loss of motion. Disorders of forearm or wrist connections result in weakness of forearm rotation, or instability and pain of the DRUJ; motion may remain full in these conditions and is limited by pain, mostly.

Nonsurgical treatment of DRUJ disorders is often successful; it includes various degrees of immobilization or antiinflammatory medication. When surgery is necessary, arthroscopy can help resolve many problems, such as TFC tear or synovitis. Many creative solutions were also developed to deal with these disorders, even before wrist arthroscopy became commonplace (**Table 1**).

Soft tissue reconstructive procedures are used primarily to stabilize the joint or dislocating ECU tendon. Ulna shortening may be used to alleviate ulnar impingement problems.[3] Destructive procedures are common for this joint. They include partial or total resection of the ulnar head or a combination of fusion and resection (Sauvé-Kapandji), with mixed results.[4–8] Early attempts at prosthetic replacement with a silicone spacer did

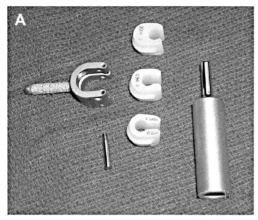
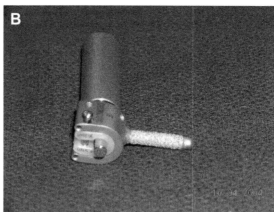
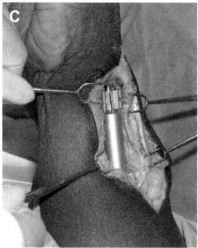

Fig. 18. (A) Wehbe mark 3 total DRUJ arthroplasty (2004). Collar was designed to fit over the retained stem in case 1. Sigmoid notch radial component includes a metallic base, 3 different size inserts to accommodate various DRUJ distances, and a lock pin. (B) Semiconstrained prosthesis assembled. (C) Semiconstrained prosthesis implanted in patient (*radiographs shown in* **Fig. 6**). (*Courtesy of* Pennsylvania Hand Center, Bryn Mawr, PA, USA; with permission.)

not withstand the test of time.[9] The ultimate salvage remains a radioulnar fusion, resulting in a 1-bone forearm, thus eliminating all forearm rotation, with predictable limitations in function.[10–12]

Prosthetic DRUJ replacement was introduced for the treatment of unstable or painful joints, because other procedures failed to provide patients with lasting relief.[13–15] Short-term results are just now being published.[16,17] Combined wrist-DRUJ prostheses have been tried, but do not seem to have withstood the test of time.[18] Most studies on the basic science of prosthetic

Table 1
Common causes of DRUJ-induced pain

	Stabilization	Resection	Shortening	Prosthesis
TFC tear		✔	✔	
Ulnar impaction		✔	✔	
Synovitis	✔	✔	✔	
Incongruity		✔	✔	✔
Degenerative joint disease		✔	✔	✔
Instability	✔	✔	✔	✔

arthroplasty of the DRUJ did not come until after implants in that joint had been in clinical use for many years.[19–24]

Prosthetic arthroplasty needs to approximate normal anatomy, which can be easily obtained from cadaver studies or examination of normal radiographs (**Fig. 19**). Prosthetic arthroplasty also introduces man-made materials into the body. Lessons learnt from other joints, such as the hip and shoulder, could make one leery of embarking on the development of a prosthesis for the DRUJ. Metal-on-bone and metal-on-metal prostheses have a poor track record.[25–28] Metal-on-polyethylene implants seem to be better tolerated, and cementing techniques (or lack of) can also be significant factors in outcome.[29] It is likely that the pain in the patient in case 1 was caused by metal-on-bone erosion. The second patient had no pain because, most likely, little or no motion occurred at the DRUJ and most of her motion took place inside the ulna shaft. The ideal DRUJ implant design would thus include either no motion of metal on articular cartilage, or metal on polyethylene. Lest we become complacent about the choice of materials, we have to be reminded of allergic reactions to metal or other components, as seen in case 1.[30]

The first DRUJ design was initially implanted in 1988 and was presented at the American Society for Surgery of the Hand in 1992.[15,31,32] Other attempts at prosthetic replacement of the DRUJ have been reported since; some had constrained designs, and others unconstrained. The constrained design purports to provide stability to the DRUJ, in addition to the resurfacing.

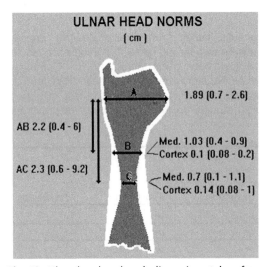

Fig. 19. Ulnar head and neck dimensions taken from radiographs of 20 normal radiographs. (*Courtesy of* Pennsylvania Hand Center, Bryn Mawr, PA, USA; with permission.)

Kapandji[14] designed a total DRUJ replacement in 1989. He implanted this in 2 patients; one replacement failed because of loosening of the radial component within 5 months, and the second patient was doing well at 10 months, except for weakness of grip.

Herbert[33] designed in 1997 an implant with a ceramic ulnar head and porous stem. A multicenter study of 23 patients with this prosthesis was published in 2000, with a follow-up of 10 to 43 months. These patients improved from their preoperative condition, but had residual pain, limitation of motion, and weakness of grip.[34] In a more recent update, with 57 patients and a mean follow-up of 38 months, the results seem unchanged, with loosening of the implant in 1 patient.[16]

A search of US and Canadian patents revealed the first DRUJ prosthesis to have been recorded in 1999, on behalf of Scheker (**Table 2**).[35] This implant consists of a long stem for the ulna and a radial component that is attached to the sigmoid notch with screws. Cooney and colleagues[36] at Mayo Clinic registered a hemiprosthesis in 2001, with a metallic ulnar head that articulates on its metallic stem. This hemiprosthesis was followed by Hubach and colleagues[37] with a combined wrist-DRUJ prosthesis in 2002. A resurfacing implant was recorded in 2004 for Kopylov and colleagues.[38] That implant seems to require minimal resection of the DRUJ. Taylor and colleagues[39] obtained a Canadian patent in 2005 for a hemiarthroplasty that incorporates an eccentric ulnar head. More recently, in 2007, Cooney and colleagues[40] obtained a patent for a sigmoid notch component.

Scheker[41] published in 2001 his experience with a constrained total DRUJ prosthesis in 23 patients. Followed up to 40 months (mean 15 months), these patients all did well, and apparently none had any complications.

The Mayo implant allows metal-to-bone contact. The ulnar head is anchored with a suture to the wrist-carpus mass, so most of the motion probably occurs at the prosthetic metal-on-metal interface, within the ulnar head. As a result, this implant may be less likely to cause problems with pain from the sigmoid notch, but the long-term effects of metal-on-metal wear are still not known. The use of this prosthesis was subsequently validated in a cadaver study.[42] More recent results on 19 wrists with more than 2 years of follow-up included 3 failures; the remainder improved in pain scores (although all seemed to have some residual pain), but there was no improvement in range of motion or strength.[30]

I could not find any reports on the use of the Hubach combined wrist-DRUJ prosthesis. This is

Table 2
Patented DRUJ prostheses

Patent Date	Filing Date	Inventors	Patent Holders	Patent Number
September 14, 1999	December 31, 1997	Scheker[35]	Avanta Orthopedics	US 5,951,604
October 16, 2001	August 30, 2000	Cooney et al[36]	Mayo Foundation	US 6,302,915 B1
November 26, 2002	July 6, 1999	Hubach et al[37]	Schaefer micomed	US 6,485,520 B1
November 9, 2004	September 20, 2002	Kopylov et al[38]	Ascension Orthopedics	US 6,814,757 B2
July 20, 2005	February 5, 2004	Taylor et al[39]	Wright Medical	CA 2513917
January 9, 2007	December 1, 2004	Cooney et al[40]	Mayo Foundation	US 7,160,331 B2

See text for References and description.

a constrained prosthesis in which the distal ulna articulates with the distal radius wrist plate.[37] No reports could be found either for Kopylov resurfacing implants; that sigmoid notch and ulnar head cap were designed for use individually or in combination.[38]

The Taylor implant is similar to the Mayo implant, the major difference being the asymmetric shape of the ulnar head component.[39] No clinical studies could be found on this implant either, although in vitro performance seemed promising.[43] The latest offering is the Mayo sigmoid notch implant, but again no long-term clinical studies have been published to support its use.[40]

There had been, until recently, only 1 option for salvage after multiple attempts at reconstruction resulting in a very short ulna: the 1-bone forearm.

This treatment may be a good option for the patient with normal shoulder, elbow, and wrist, who can compensate for loss of forearm rotation. Even then, such a patient has a great deal of difficulty with some activities of daily living.

DRUJ prosthetic replacement is still in its infancy, and any degree of failure does not negate the rewards of success. Failure rates have been high for most joints and the wrist in particular. The development of better prostheses and surgical techniques should continue to improve outcome.

Many designs have been offered, covering a spectrum of designs (**Table 3**). Hemiarthroplasties have the potential of causing pain, in the long-term, as a result of the friction of an intact articular surface against plastic or metal. A recent report had a 30% failure rate in DRUJ arthroplasty,

Table 3
DRUJ prostheses design

Unconstrained (Hemiarthroplasty)	Constrained	Semiconstrained
Wehbe (1988)[a]	Kapandji (1989)[b]	
Wehbe (1992)[c]		
Herbert (1995)[d]	Scheker (1997)[e]	
Cooney et al (2000)[f]		
Kopylov et al (2002)[g]	Hubach et al (1999)[h]	
King (2003)[i]		Wehbe (2004)[j]
Ascension (2006)[k]		
Cooney et al (2007)[l]		

[a] Wehbe Mark 1 Design. Custom Implant, Biomet, Warsaw, IN.
[b] Custom Implant, Kapandji AI, Longjumeau, France.
[c] Wehbe Mark 2 Design. Custom Implant, Biomet, Warsaw, IN.
[d] Orthosurgical Implants, Miami, FL.
[e] Aptis Medical, LLC, Louisville, KY.
[f] uHead, Small Bone Innovations, Morrisville, PA.
[g] Ascension Orthopedics, Austin, TX.
[h] Schaefer micomed, Goppingen, Denmark.
[i] E-Centrix, Wright Medical Technology, Arlington, TN.
[j] Wehbe Mark 3 Design. Custom Implant, Biomet, Warsaw, IN.
[k] First Choice DRUJ System, Ascension Orthopedics, Austin, TX.
[l] Mayo Design, Small Bone Innovations, Morrisville, PA.

with a 4.5-year follow-up.[44] A total joint replacement carries its own problems, mostly with potential incongruency of components, as well as friction between man-made materials. Nonconstrained systems have an inherent risk of instability, and constrained systems a risk of loosening.

More than a decade ago, Julio Taleisnik stated: "I am for the most part, very pleased with the forms of treatment that we have at present. I am not sure that a prosthesis would be a reliable long-term answer to the problem."[45] With the recent surge of interest in prosthetic replacement of the DRUJ, we may be optimistic that we will eventually achieve long-term successful implantation with a variety of options that allow us to select the best implant for each particular patient. To achieve this goal, we must learn from the trials and tribulations of the past.

REFERENCES

1. Buck-Gramcko D. On the priorities of publication of some operative procedures on the distal end of the ulna. J Hand Surg 1990;15B:416–20.
2. Bieber JB, Linscheid RL, Bobyns JH, et al. Failed distal ulna resections. J Hand Surg 1988;13A:193–200.
3. Chidgey LK. The distal radio-ulnar joints: problems and solutions. J Am Acad Orthop Surg 1995;3:95–109.
4. Bowers WH. Distal radio-ulnar joint arthroplasty: the hemiresection-interposition technique. J Hand Surg 1985;10A:169–78.
5. Inagaki H, Nakamura R, Horii E, et al. Symptoms and radiographic findings in the proximal and distal ulnar stumps after Sauvé-Kapandji procedure for treatment of chronic derangement of the distal radio-ulnar joint. J Hand Surg 2006;31A:780–4.
6. Newmeyer WL, Green DP. Rupture of digital extensor tendon following distal ulnar resection. J Bone Joint Surg Am 1982;64A:178–82.
7. Watson HK, Ryu J, Burgess RC. Matched distal ulnar resection. J Hand Surg 1986;11A:812–7.
8. Wolfe SW, Mih AD, Culp RW, et al. Wide excision of the distal ulna: a multicenter case study. J Hand Surg 1998;23A:222–8.
9. McMurtry RY, Paley D, Marks P, et al. A critical analysis of Swanson ulnar head replacement arthroplasty: rheumatoid versus nonrheumatoid. J Hand Surg 1990;15A:224–31.
10. Lee SJ, Jazrawi LM, Ong BC, et al. Long-term follow-up of the one-bone forearm procedure. Am J Orthop 2000;29:969–72.
11. Peterson CA, Maki S, Wood MB. Clinical results of the one-bone forearm. J Hand Surg 1995;20A:609–18.
12. Schneider LH, Imbriglia JE. Radio-ulnar joint fusion for distal radio-ulnar joint instability. Hand Clin 1991;7:391–5.
13. Fernandez DL, Joneschild ES, Abella DM. Treatment of failed Sauvé-Kapandji procedures with a spherical ulnar head prosthesis. Clin Orthop Relat Res 2006; 445:100–7.
14. Kapandji AI. Distal radio-ulnar prosthesis. Ann Chir Main Memb Super 1992;11:320–32.
15. Wehbé MA. Pitfall of distal radio-ulnar joint injuries. Jefferson Orthop J 1992;21:30–3.
16. van Schoonhoven J, Herbert TJ, Fernandez DL, et al. Ulnar head prosthesis. Orthopade 2003;32: 809–15.
17. Willis AA, Berger RA, Cooney WP. Arthroplasty of the distal radio-ulnar joint using a new ulnar head endoprosthesis: preliminary report. J Hand Surg 2007; 32A:177–89.
18. Bodell LS, Leonard L. Wrist arthroplasty. In: Berger RA, Weiss AP, editors. Hand surgery. Philadelphia: Lippincott; 2004. p. 1339–94.
19. Austman RL, Beaton BJ, Quenneville CE, et al. The effect of distal ulnar implant stem material and length on bone strains. J Hand Surg 2007;32A: 848–54.
20. Gordon KD, Roth SE, Dunning CE, et al. An anthropometric study of the distal ulna: implications for implant design. J Hand Surg 2002;27A:57–60.
21. Gordon KD, Kedgley AE, Ferreira LM, et al. Design and implementation of an instrumented ulnar head prosthesis to measure loads in vitro. J Biomech 2006;39:1335–41.
22. King GJ, McMurtry RY, Rubenstein JD, et al. Kinematics of the distal radio-ulnar joint. J Hand Surg 1986;11A:798–804.
23. Masaoka S, Longsworth SH, Werner FW, et al. Biomechanical analysis of two ulnar head prostheses. J Hand Surg 2002;27A:845–53.
24. Sauerbier MH, Fujita M, Neale PG, et al. Dynamic radio-ulnar convergence after Darrach operation, soft tissue stabilizing operations of the distal ulna and ulnar head prosthesis implantation–an experimental biomechanical study. Unfallchirurg 2002; 105:688–98.
25. Huo MH, Dumont GD, Knight JR, et al. What's new in total hip arthroplasty. J Bone Joint Surg Am 2011;93: 1944–50.
26. Isaac GH, Thompson J, Williams S, et al. Metal-on-metal bearings surfaces: materials, manufacture, design, optimization, and alternatives. Proc Inst Mech Eng 2006;220:119–33.
27. Merritt K, Rodrigo JJ. Immune response to synthetic materials. Sensitization of patients receiving orthopaedic implants. Clin Orthop Relat Res 1996;326: 71–9.
28. Savarino L, Granchi D, Ciapetti G, et al. Ion release inpatients with metal-on-metal hip bearings in total joint replacement: a comparison with metal-on-polyethylene bearings. J Biomed Mater Res 2002; 63:467–74.

29. Sanchez-Sotelo J, Berry DJ, Harmsen S. Long-term results of use of a collared matte-finished femoral component fixed with second-generation cementing techniques. J Bone Joint Surg Am 2002;84:1636–41.

30. Nasser S. Orthopedic metal immune hypersensitivity. Orthopedics 2007;30:89–91.

31. Wehbé MA. Pitfalls of radio-ulnar joint injuries. Jefferson Orthopaedic Society Annual Meeting. Philadelphia, November 15, 1991.

32. Wehbé MA. Pitfalls of distal radio-ulnar joint surgery, Symposium, American Society for Surgery of the Hand Annual Meeting. Phoenix, November 13, 1992.

33. van Schoonhoven J, Herbert TJ, Krimmer H. New concepts for endoprostheses of the distal radio-ulnar joint. Handchir Mikrochir Plast Chir 1998;30: 387–92.

34. van Schoonhoven J, Fernandez DL, Bowers WH, et al. Salvage of failed resection arthroplasties of the distal radio-ulnar joint using a new ulnar head prosthesis. J Hand Surg 2000;25A:438–46.

35. Scheker LR. Distal radio-ulnar joint prosthesis. United States Patent Number 5,951,604. 1999.

36. Cooney WP, Berger RA, Linscheid RL, et al. Ulnar implant system. United States Patent Number 6,302,915 B1. 2001.

37. Hubach PC, Schafer B, Trauwein T. Wrist prosthesis. United States Patent Number 6,485,520 B1. 2002.

38. Kopylov P, Tagil L, Ogilvie WF. Joint surface replacement of the distal radio-ulnar joint. United States Patent Number 6,814,757 B2. 2004.

39. Taylor A, Patterson SD, Hanson S, et al. Articulating implant system. Canada Patent Number 2513917. 2005.

40. Cooney WP, Berger RA, Leibel DA. Sigmoid notch implant. United States Patent Number 7,160,331 B2. 2007.

41. Scheker LR, Babb BA, Killion PE. Distal ulnar prosthetic replacement. Orthop Clin North Am 2001;32: 365–76.

42. Sauerbier M, Hahn ME, Masaki F, et al. Analysis of dynamic distal radio-ulnar convergence after ulnar head resection and endoprosthesis implantation. J Hand Surg 2002;27A:425–34.

43. Gordon KD, Dunning CE, Johnson JA, et al. Kinematics of ulnar head arthroplasty. J Hand Surg 2003;28B:551–8.

44. Kakar S, Swann RP, Perry KI, et al. Functional and radiographic outcomes following distal ulnar implant arthroplasty. J Hand Surg 2012;37A:1364–71.

45. Taleisnik J. Letter to the author, March 9 1993.

Implant Arthroplasty for Treatment of Ulnar Head Resection–Related Instability

Richard A. Berger, MD, PhD

KEYWORDS

• Ulnar head arthroplasty • Distal radioulnar joint • Salvage

KEY POINTS

- The ulnar head serves as a cantilever, in concert with the flare of the distal radius metaphysis, to keep the radius and ulna separated and the stabilizing structures of the distal forearm joint under tension.
- The ulnar head serves as a support for the ulnar side of the wrist, typically transmitting 20% of the longitudinal load applied across the wrist.
- It serves as the boney foundation for the fibro-osseous tunnel of the tendon of the extensor carpi ulnaris, keeping it channeled for optimal performance. There may be more functions that we simply are not aware of yet.

What are the possible functions of the ulnar head? It serves as the ulnar component in the distal radioulnar joint. As such, it participates in the kinematic guidance of the radius–wrist–hand unit as it rotates and translates about the fixed ulna. The ulnar head serves as a cantilever, in concert with the flare of the distal radius metaphysis, to keep the radius and ulna separated and the stabilizing structures of the distal forearm joint under tension. The ulnar head serves as a support for the ulnar side of the wrist, typically transmitting 20% of the longitudinal load applied across the wrist.[1] It serves as an attachment for the stabilizers of the distal radioulnar joint as well as the ulnocarpal joint. It serves as the boney foundation for the fibro-osseous tunnel of the tendon of the extensor carpi ulnaris, keeping it channeled for optimal performance. There may be more functions that we simply are not aware of yet. We know that these functions are valid because of the effects observed when the ulnar head is excised for the treatment of mechanical impingement or painful arthrosis. This article reviews treatment options for such conditions, and the progressive efforts to maintain the functions of the ulnar head despite having it resected in part or in full.

MECHANICS STUDIES

Forearm rotation occurs about nonfixed axes of rotation. The motions of the proximal and distal radioulnar joints are the same, because the radius and ulna are rigid bodies. Simply stated, the radius–wrist–hand unit "pivots" about the ulna, rotationally anchored at the proximal radioulnar joint. The axes of rotation penetrate the radial head at its geometric center. They pass obliquely distally to exit through the ulnar head at the fovea. The penetration points translate reciprocally through pronation and supination, such that they are more anterior in pronation and more posterior in supination. This translation of the location of the axes of

Disclosure: See last page of the article.
Division of Hand Surgery, Orthopedic Surgery, Mayo Clinic, 200 1st Street Southwest, Rochester, MN 55905, USA
E-mail address: berger.richard@mayo.edu

Hand Clin 29 (2013) 103–111
http://dx.doi.org/10.1016/j.hcl.2012.08.028
0749-0712/13/$ – see front matter © 2013 Elsevier Inc. All rights reserved

hand.theclinics.com

rotation defines the actual translation of the radius relative to the ulnar head, which augments the range of rotation to provide up to 180° of forearm rotation. This is allowed because of different radii of curvature for the concave sigmoid notch and the convex ulnar head. With the radius of curvature of the ulnar head smaller than that of the sigmoid notch, translation is allowed in addition to rotation. Without this action, the pivot of the radius is dramatically reduced and thus the range of forearm rotation is proportionately reduced. We have learned from laboratory studies that the ulnar head itself contributes to the constraint of the distal radioulnar joint by approximately 20%.[2] Resecting the ulnar head in a dynamic, cadaver-based, mechanical simulator demonstrated "extreme instability" with movement of the radius toward the ulna.[3] Taking this further, attempts to regain stability after resecting the ulnar head with either interposition of the pronator quadratus or performing a tenodesis with the tendons of flexor and extensor carpi ulnaris failed to reduce radioulnar convergence.[4] Finally, it was also demonstrated that resecting the ulnar head reduces torque resistance strength of the forearm.[5]

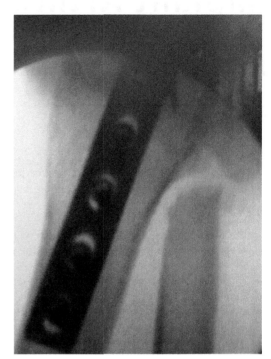

Fig. 1. Posterioranterior radiograph of a wrist after ulnar head resection, demonstrating "convergence instability."

CLINICAL OUTCOMES OF DARRACH AND SAUVE-KAPANDJI

Despite the intuitive sense that resecting the ulnar head would result in instability between the radius and ulna and despite the laboratory studies highlighted, numerous reports have been published about the clinical outcomes after resection of the ulnar head, many of which show favorable outcomes, noting increase range of motion, decreased pain, and improvement in grip strength despite radiographic evidence of radioulnar convergence (**Fig. 1**).[6–8] Others, however, hold that radioulnar convergence is clinically important and leads to suboptimal results. Scheker[9] has demonstrated an easy way to radiograph convergence by taking a cross-table posterioranterior radiograph with the patient holding onto a 5-pound weight. Although normative torque strengths have been measured, there have not been any published investigations about the effect of ulnar head resection on forearm torque strength.[10] Considering the goals of resection arthroplasty of the distal ulna for providing pain relief from arthrosis involving the ulnar head or sigmoid notch, "unlocking" forearm rotation in cases of dislocated or subluxed distal radioulnar joint after a displaced distal radius fracture, or relieving pressure on adjacent neurovascular structured from developmental deformities like Madelung's disorder, a successful outcome related to these specific goals has a reasonable chance of occurring, given the appropriate levels of activities and expectations of the patient. The less demanding and more sedentary the patient's lifestyle is, the more likely the instability problems associated with resection of the ulnar head will be. And under these circumstances, the more likely soft tissue-based interposition procedures will provide a satisfactory outcome.[11–13]

IMPLANT ARTHROPLASTY

In an attempt to recreate the stabilizing properties of the native ulnar head after resection, implantation of artificial ulnar heads has been introduced, beginning in 1973 with the introduction of a silicone rubber implant.[14] These 1-piece implants were demonstrated to provide relieve in patients experiencing posttraumatic radioulnar instability after ulnar head resection, with up to 70% of patients in 1 study experiencing good or excellent results an average of 44 months after implantation.[15] This same study, however, reveals tilting of the implant in 40% and implant fractures in 15%. In another study, implant breakage or migration was seen in 63% of 45 wrists studied with histologic demonstration of silicone synovitis in patients requiring implant removal.[16] These authors concluded that silicone rubber ulnar head prostheses are contraindicated, confirmed by others[17]; indeed, they are no longer manufactured.

Recognizing the shortcomings of the silicone rubber implants, Herbert designed a modular system with a ceramic ulnar head fitting onto a metallic stem inserted into the ulna that was released onto the market in 1995.[18] The head is capable of rotating on the stem as the radius dynamically rotates around the ulna. The developer emphasizes that success comes not only from appropriate implantation of the device, but also from regaining soft-tissue stability and that the implant is seated, a theme that follows subsequent implant development. Initial results at an average of 27 months demonstrated stability and marked symptomatic improvement in patients. These results have stood up to time with a recent long-term, follow-up publication evaluating patients up to 11 years after implantation. All clinical parameters remained significantly improved from preoperative assessments, and radiographs demonstrated no stem loosening.[19] This device has also been reported as a salvage technique for failed Sauve-Kapandji procedures in 3 patients with good results at up to 22 months after implantation.[20]

Soon after the release of the Herbert implant, other implants became available from several manufacturers. Each was developed as a modular system, with different sized head dimensions and stem dimensions (**Fig. 2**). Each procedure depends on soft-tissue stabilization through repair, reefing, or reconstruction of the distal radioulnar joint capsule. Laboratory studies using a cadaver-based dynamic simulator demonstrated significant restoration of loads and kinematics toward normal after implantation of an ulnar head metallic prosthesis compared with resection of the ulnar head.[5] This also included an observation that resistance to torque improved significantly after implantation. The only study specifically comparing 2 different implant systems was performed in the laboratory, where the forearm rotation, diastasis between the radius and ulna, and dorsal/palmar subluxation were measured in varying forearm positions.[21] It was discovered that both implant systems maintained near-normal biomechanics of the distal radioulnar joint compared with the unpredictable mechanics after ulnar head resection. Initial clinical results of ulnar head replacement with a metallic implant demonstrated 50% pain improvement and a 3-fold patient satisfaction result 2 years after implantation.[22] A recent publication evaluating patients at a longer follow-up demonstrated 83% survival at 6 years, but 30% of patients required some additional procedure after the initial procedure. Risk factors for failure included a history of previous surgery, use of an extension collar, and loosening of the stem.[23] In this author's experience, there is an increased risk of loosening in patients with a complete wrist arthrodesis (**Fig. 3**). Two implant systems were evaluated clinically by a single surgeon and published. No differences between the 2 systems were detected, but both systems resulted in good outcomes, regardless of whether the implantation was performed at the time of ulnar head resection or as a revision procedure.[24] A suggested postoperative rehabilitation protocol has been published that progressively advances activities in 2-week increments through 12 weeks, with a well-defined "stop point" if issues occur with the patient's progress.[25]

Recently, an implant was introduced that is made of pyrocarbon and is designed to replace only the articular "seat" of the ulna, leaving the styloid process and perhaps even the foveal attachment of the triangular fibrocartilage complex intact, thus potentially improving stability of the distal radioulnar joint. A radiographic study using cadaver specimens demonstrated that this implant can closely recreate the articular anatomy of the ulnar head without extensive soft-tissue dissection, thus theoretically improving stability.[26] Clinically, a small series studying 3 patients at an average of 11 months after implantation of this device demonstrated minimal discomfort, functional forearm motion (65° supination and 70° pronation), and that all patients could lift 4-kg of load throughout the forearm range of motion.[27]

A linked prosthesis is designed to provide intrinsic stability by "connecting" radial and ulnar prosthetic components through a movable linkage.[9] This topic is beyond the scope of this article, but is covered in subsequently in this volume.

LESSONS LEARNED TO DATE

The greatest lesson for all surgeons dealing with the painful distal radioulnar joint is to do all we can to maintain the ulnar head in place as long as possible. As noted in the introduction, the ulnar

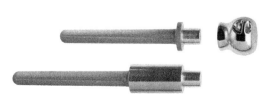

Fig. 2. Modular ulnar head implant arthroplasty. The head and stem are manufactured in different sizes, but a universal coupling allows for interchanges of different-sized components.

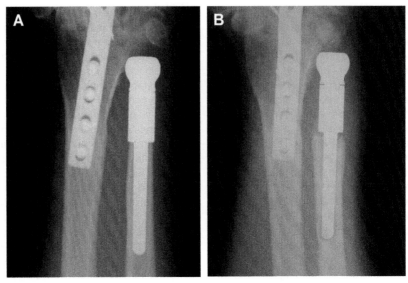

Fig. 3. Posterioranterior radiographs of an ulnar head implant arthroplasty in a patient with a preexisting total wrist fusion (*A*) immediately postoperatively. (*B*) At 1 year postoperatively. Note the lucency around the stem of the implant, the hypertrophic growth of bone near the implant collar, and the tilt of the implant, all indicating loosening.

head serves many purposes, all of which are at risk if it is resected, either entirely or partially, or if its function is disconnected from the forearm joint through a distal arthrodesis and creation of a more proximal pseudoarthrosis. Resecting the ulnar head when pain alone is the principle finding should be gravely contemplated. Once the ulnar head is gone, it cannot be replaced to the original design specification, even with modern implants.

Indications

Indications for implant arthroplasty after resection of the ulnar head are principally related to painful instability. This can be either primary at the time of ulnar head resection, or secondary as a postoperative complaint. The instability can be 3 dimensional, but convergence instability is the most painful and is usually what brings the patient to their surgeon. Anteroposterior instability can be unsettling to the patient, and may be related to their sense of weakness. Implant arthroplasty shows significant advantages over soft-tissue stabilization procedures in these patients, and should be considered as a core indication.

Absolute Contraindications

As with any implant, an active infection in the surgical site is an absolute contraindication to proceeding with implant surgery. Unless special circumstances are defined, remote infections should also be considered contraindications to implant arthroplasty. Patients with deficient motors

for forearm rotation are contraindicated, whether from primarily neurologic causes, traumatic loss, or scar tissue impeding tendon excursion. These implants must have adequate soft-tissue coverage to provide a functional range of motion, stability, and pain relief. Any compromise in the soft tissues available for stabilization and coverage needs to be addressed before implantation of the device. And because these devices all depend on soft-tissue stability, in addition to the presence of the implant itself, active inflammatory arthropathy of the wrist or distal radioulnar joint should be well-controlled medically, surgically, or through a combined approach before proceeding with implant arthroplasty.

Relative Contraindications

Significant instability detected clinically in patients undergoing consideration for implant arthroplasty must be evaluated before proceeding. If the patient demonstrates instability with their native ulnar head, they will likely demonstrate instability with an implant arthroplasty, unless something changes. The instability may be the result of erosions of the ulnar head, such as in prior episodes of inflammatory arthropathy. This may be resolved with the implantation of an appropriately sized ulnar head implant, but be aware that the capsular soft tissues may have been adversely affect, requiring tightening or reconstruction. There may be deficiencies of the sigmoid notch, reducing its ability to "capture" the ulnar head.

This may prompt the need for a sigmoid notch implant in addition to the ulnar head implant. It may also raise considerations for a linked implant, which brings its own stability into the joint.

Angular malalignment of the sigmoid notch relative to the ulna and the axis of rotation is a relative contraindication for implant arthroplasty of the ulnar head (**Fig. 4**). There are no absolute upper and lower limits of tolerance for this malalignment; some patients are stable with 30° of dorsal angulation of the distal radius after a fracture, whereas others are unstable with 10° of angular change. Some cases of instability are the results of healed radius or ulna fractures in childhood that have become unstable over time owing to continued longitudinal growth of the affected bone. The surgeon needs to be diligent about looking for bony causes of joint instability and always use comparison imaging of the contralateral extremity. If malalignment is detected or suspected, it should be addressed before implantation of an ulnar head replacement – either at the same setting or in a staged fashion.

Residual Instability

Once an implant is in place, this author always recommend testing the stability of the forearm by anteriorly and posteriorly stressing the distal radioulnar joint throughout the range of pronation and supination. If subluxation occurs, it should be addressed at the time of surgery. Instability can also occur gradually over time postoperatively. Regardless of when it occurs, once it is detected, efforts should be made to identify the cause(s) and develop a plan for correction. The principal causes of instability in my experience are soft tissue insufficiency, sigmoid notch insufficiency, and malalignment of the sigmoid notch.

Soft-tissue insufficiency may involve deficiency of the dorsal and palmar radioulnar ligaments, attenuation of the distal radioulnar joint capsule, loss of integrity of the ulnocarpal ligaments, or any combination of these factors. When the ulnar head is resected entirely, it by default temporarily disrupts the distal radioulnar ligaments. Although the ligaments cannot heal back into the implant, they can be incorporated into the capsular closure to provide at least some stabilizing effect. At least 1 implant system has provisions for temporarily stabilizing the ligaments directly to the implant (**Fig. 5**).

Sigmoid notch insufficiency can be detected with axial imaging such as computed tomography or magnetic resonance imaging preoperatively. Although not explicitly promoted in the operative techniques of the implants, the author has found this useful, especially when imaging is compared between both extremities. If there is excessive dorsal angulation of the sigmoid notch, the author does revise the surgical plan to a linked implant, owing to concerns about the ease of volar subluxation of the radius through the deficient sigmoid notch. The author has not found wedge notchplasty effective under these circumstances. There may be a role for using a sigmoid notch implant matched to the ulnar head implant to regain the appropriate orientation of the articulation (**Fig. 6**).

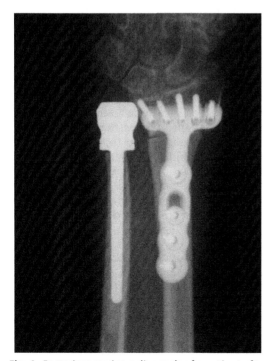

Fig. 4. Posterioranterior radiograph of a patient after ulnar head implant arthroplasty. A corrective osteotomy of the distal radius was performed to normalize the alignment of the sigmoid notch for the implant.

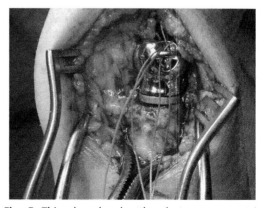

Fig. 5. This ulnar head arthroplasty component is designed to allow temporary suture fixation of the joint capsule to augment stability.

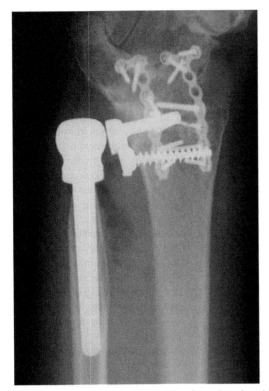

Fig. 6. Posterioranterior radiograph of an ulnar head implant arthroplasty, complemented by a sigmoid notch component.

Sigmoid notch orientation, as noted, can present a significant challenge for maintaining stability.[28] Numerous causes of abnormal orientation of the sigmoid notch can be encountered, including developmental causes such as Madelung's deformity, fractures in adulthood that are inadequately reduced and maintained, or even fractures of the radius or ulna before skeletal maturity that subsequently create a progressively worsening problem with growth. After comparing x-rays with the contralateral forearm and wrist, if an angular malalignment is detected, consideration for correcting it through an osteotomy with internal fixation should be made before implantation of the ulnar head replacement.

Intraoperative efforts to improve stability can be achieved in several ways. First, each implant system has surgical techniques that describe the importance of raising appropriate fascial and capsular flaps to be used in stabilizing the implant at closure. These techniques are important to follow. If instability is detected after the implant is seated, taking the modular ulnar head off and replacing it with a larger size often solves the problem. Some authors have reported difficulty in uncoupling the ulnar head from the stem, but

instrumentation improvements have largely resolved this issue.[29] Implantation of a matched sigmoid notch component can improve stability by (1) creating a deeper concave surface for the ulnar head to articulate with and (2) increasing the separation between the radius and ulna, thus increasing the tension on the soft-tissue stabilizers. There are no large-scale, clinical series published with this technique, so experience in rare and anecdotal. Osteoplasty of the sigmoid notch has been advocated by Adams as a technique to deepen the curvature of the sigmoid notch, but its application to implant arthroplasty has not been published.[30]

After the implantation procedure is completed and the patient is pacing through their rehabilitation steps, instability may develop, albeit uncommonly. If it does, the root cause of the instability must be determined as soon as possible. If it is instability discovered immediately after the procedure, it is possible that altering the position of forearm immobilization will resolve the instability, as long as the window of healing opportunity is still open. Placing the forearm in supination for volar displacement of the radius relative to the ulna, or vice versa into pronation for dorsal displacement, may resolve the issue, but one should make all efforts to ensure that a diastasis has not occurred between the radius and ulna, which will not resolve with time and immobilization. These patients require additional surgery.

Additional staged procedures to stabilize the radius to the ulna may include the use of a distally based brachioradialis tendon drawn volarly to the ulnar neck or a distally based strip of flexor carpi ulnaris tendon, wrapped around the ulnar neck (**Fig. 7**).[31] If capsular insufficiency is suspected, creation of a capsule reconstruction with allograft facial lata has been a useful technique. The fascial strip is anchored to the volar rim of the sigmoid notch with bone anchors, and the strip is drawn dorsally, deep to the extensor carpi ulnaris tendon, and secured to the dorsal rim of the sigmoid notch, under the maximum tendon (**Fig. 8**).

Subsidence

Subsidence can occur with the hardness of the ulnar implant is significantly greater than the hardness of the radius. This can be a worrisome scenario, because progressive subsidence can undermine the support for the lunate fossa (**Fig. 9**). Patients particularly at risk for this are those being revised from a Sauve-Kapandji procedure where the arthrodesed ulnar head is resected, patients with severe osteopenia, and those who have undergone any burring of the

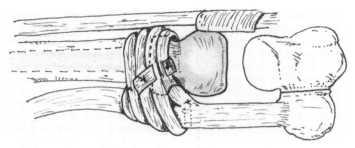

Fig. 7. Drawing of a technique using a distally based strip of flexor carpi ulnaris wrapped around the neck of an ulnar head implant arthroplasty to augment stability.

sigmoid notch to the level of exposing cancellous bone for the purpose of deepening its curvature. If underlying cancellous bone is exposed to the ulnar head implant, either adding a sigmoid notch component or converting to a linked total distal radioulnar implant is advised.

Loosening

Loosening of any implant, regardless of location, can be significantly problematic. Fortunately, loosening of currently available ulnar head implants is rare. It is not uncommon to have some degree of bony resorption just proximal to the ulnar head, presumably owing to stress shielding. This is not loosening of the implant and can be ignored, as long as it is not progressive and does not threaten the stability of the implant. In this author's experience using a metallic ulnar head, nearly all occurrences of stem loosening have occurred in association with a complete wrist arthrodesis. The underlying mechanism is not known, but it may have something to do with torque transmission. In an intact wrist, each joint between the metacarpals and carpal bones, between the carpal bones, and between the carpus and the forearm bones pronates and supinates to some extent, thus theoretically absorbs torque forces. With a complete wrist arthrodesis, torque transmission across the en bloc carpus straight to the implant occurs. If the head of the implant is incapable of rotating on the stem, that torque is transmitted to the stem/bone interface. In this manner, it is possible that stem loosening can occur. If such loosening occurs, even if currently asymptomatic, planning for revision surgery should be initiated.

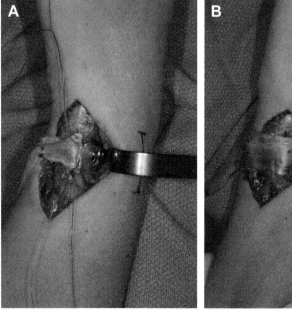
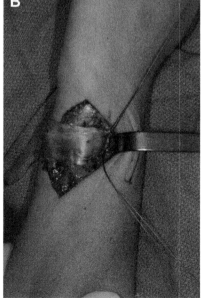

Fig. 8. The distal radioulnar joint capsule can be reconstructed with a strip of allograft fascia lata. It is first secured to the volar rim of the radius with bone anchors (*A*) and then drawn dorsally (*B*), deep to the tendon of extensor carpi ulnaris and secured with sutures to the dorsal rim of the sigmoid notch.

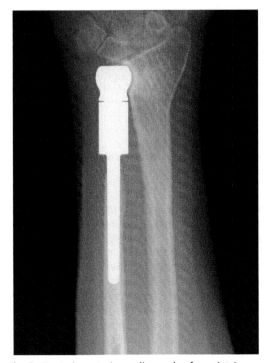

Fig. 9. Posterioranterior radiograph of a wrist 4 years after conversion of a Sauve-Kapandji procedure to an ulnar head implant arthroplasty. Note the subsidence of the implant into the radius, undermining the support for the lunate fossa.

Other causes of loosening to consider would be indolent infection and metal allergy. Efforts to rule out infection would include serology, scintigraphy, and open tissue acquisition for histopathology and cultures. Metal allergy can be assessed through skin testing with metal samples.

Revision Options

If revision is necessary for any of the reasons cited, there are several options. First, simply explanting the device can be considered. It is no different than having the resection arthroplasty in the first place. If the patient does not want more involved surgery, they may be satisfied with reversion back to baseline. Converting to an interposition arthroplasty with a roll of allograft Achilles tendon may provide excellent relief. Conversion to a linked total distal radioulnar joint implant can be considered. Finally, although rarely indicated, conversion to a 1-bone forearm provides the ultimate salvage option.

SUMMARY

Resection of the ulnar head in cases of debilitating pain owing to arthrosis of the distal radioulnar joint can provide satisfying relief. However, there is mounting evidence that pain with heavier use, instability, and torque-generating weakness in more active individuals may result in less satisfying outcomes. Implant arthroplasty can provide a means to stabilize the radius to the ulna after ulnar head resection, but it requires significant attention to requisite soft tissue stabilization and alignment of the distal radius to the implant to be successful.

DISCLOSURE

The author has a financial relationship with a manufacturer regarding royalties received for the development of an ulnar head implant. To manage this conflict of interest, the author will make no treatment recommendations regarding any particular implant currently available today. Additionally, because different systems are available to surgeons around the world, I will not detail the surgical techniques. These are implant specific and the user should refer to guides provided by the manufactures.

REFERENCES

1. Werner FW, Palmer AK, Fortino MD, et al. Force transmission through the distal ulna: effect of ulnar variance, lunate fossa angulation, and radial and palmar tilt of the distal radius. J Hand Surg Am 1992;17(3):423–8.
2. Stuart PR, Berger RA, Linscheid RL, et al. The dorsopalmar stability of the distal radioulnar joint. J Hand Surg Am 2000;25(4):689–99.
3. Sauerbier M, Fujita M, Hahn ME, et al. The dynamic radioulnar convergence of the Darrach procedure and the ulnar head hemiresection interposition arthroplasty: a biomechanical study. J Hand Surg Br 2002;27(4):307–16.
4. Sauerbier M, Berger RA, Fujita M, et al. Radioulnar convergence after distal ulnar resection: mechanical performance of two commonly used soft tissue stabilizing procedures. Acta Orthop Scand 2003; 74(4):420–8.
5. Sauerbier M, Hahn ME, Fujita M, et al. Analysis of dynamic distal radioulnar convergence after ulnar head resection and endoprosthesis implantation. J Hand Surg Am 2002;27(3):425–34.
6. McKee MD, Richards RR. Dynamic radio-ulnar convergence after the Darrach procedure. J Bone Joint Surg Br 1996;78(3):413–8.
7. Tulipan DJ, Eaton RG, Eberhart RE. The Darrach procedure defended: technique redefined and long-term follow-up. J Hand Surg Am 1991;16(3):438–44.
8. Kapandji IA. The Kapandji-Sauvé operation. Its techniques and indications in non rheumatoid diseases. Ann Chir Main 1986;5(3):181–93.

9. Scheker LR. Implant arthroplasty for the distal radio-ulnar joint. J Hand Surg Am 2008;33(9):1639–44.

10. Matsuoka J, Berger RA, Berglund LJ, et al. An analysis of symmetry of torque strength of the forearm under resisted forearm rotation in normal subjects. J Hand Surg Am 2006;31(5):801–5.

11. Bowers WH. Distal radioulnar joint arthroplasty: the hemiresection-interposition technique. J Hand Surg Am 1985;10(2):169–78.

12. Greenberg JA, Sotereanos D. Achilles allograft interposition for failed Darrach distal ulna resections. Tech Hand Up Extrem Surg 2008;12(2):121–5.

13. Watson HK, Ryu JY, Burgess RC. Matched distal ulnar resection. J Hand Surg Am 1986;11(6):812–7.

14. Swanson AB. Implant arthroplasty for disabilities of the distal radioulnar joint. Use of a silicone rubber capping implant following resection of the ulnar head. Orthop Clin North Am 1973;4(2):373–82.

15. Stanley D, Herbert TJ. The Swanson ulnar head prosthesis for post-traumatic disorders of the distal radio-ulnar joint. J Hand Surg Br 1992;17:682–8.

16. Sagerman SD, Seiler JG, Fleming LL, et al. Silicone rubber distal ulnar replacement arthroplasty. J Hand Surg Br 1992;17(6):689–93.

17. Schernberg F, Gerard Y, Collin JP, et al. Arthroplasty of the rheumatoid wrist by silicone implants. Experience with forty cases. Ann Chir Main 1983; 2(1):18–26.

18. Van Schoonhoven J, Fernandez DL, Bowers WH, et al. Salvage of failed resection arthroplasties of the distal radioulnar joint using a new ulnar head prosthesis. J Hand Surg 2000;25A:438.

19. van Schoonhoven J, Mühldorfer-Fodor M, Fernandez DL, et al. Salvage of failed resection arthroplasties of the distal radioulnar joint using an ulnar head prosthesis: long-term results. J Hand Surg Am 2012;37(7):1372–80.

20. De Smet L, Peeters T. Salvage of failed Sauvé-Kapandji procedure with an ulnar head prosthesis: report of three cases. J Hand Surg Br 2003;28(3):271–3.

21. Masaoka S, Longsworth SH, Werner FW, et al. Biomechanical analysis of two ulnar head prostheses. J Hand Surg Am 2002;27(5):845–53.

22. Willis AA, Berger RA, Cooney WP 3rd. Arthroplasty of the distal radioulnar joint using a new ulnar head endoprosthesis: preliminary report. J Hand Surg Am 2007;32(2):177–89.

23. Kakar S, Swann RP, Perry KI, et al. Functional and radiographic outcomes following distal ulna implant arthroplasty. J Hand Surg Am 2012;37(7):1364–71.

24. Yen Shipley N, Dion GR, Bowers WH. Ulnar head implant arthroplasty: an intermediate term review of 1 surgeon's experience. Tech Hand Up Extrem Surg 2009;13(3):160–4.

25. Kaiser GL, Bodell LS, Berger RA. Functional outcomes after arthroplasty of the distal radioulnar joint and hand therapy: a case series. J Hand Ther 2008;21(4):398–409.

26. Conaway DA, Kuhl TL, Adams BD. Comparison of the native ulnar head and a partial ulnar head resurfacing implant. J Hand Surg Am 2009;34(6): 1056–62.

27. Garcia-Elias M. Eclypse: partial ulnar head replacement for the isolated distal radio-ulnar joint arthrosis. Tech Hand Up Extrem Surg 2007;11(1):121–8.

28. Tolat AR, Stanley JK, Trail IA. A cadaveric study of the anatomy and stability of the distal radioulnar joint in the coronal and transverse planes. J Hand Surg Br 1996;21(5):587–94.

29. Naidu SH, Radin A. Modular ulnar head decoupling force: case report. J Hand Surg Am 2009;34(6): 1063–5.

30. Adams BD. Distal radio-ulnar joint instability. In: Berger RA, Weiss AP, editors. Hand surgery. Philadelphia: Lippincott Williams and Wilkins; 2004. p. 347.

31. Burke CS, Gupta A, Buecker P. Distal ulna giant cell tumor resection with reconstruction using distal ulna prosthesis and brachioradialis wrap soft tissue stabilization. Hand (N Y) 2009;4(4):410–4.

Distal Radioulnar Joint Constrained Arthroplasty

Luis R. Scheker, MD[a,b,*], David W. Martineau, MD[a,c]

KEYWORDS

- Distal radioulnar joint ● Wrist prosthesis ● Arthroplasty ● Ulnar impingement

KEY POINTS

- The distal radioulnar joint (DRUJ) is a complex articulation that carries weight while allowing vector changes without interfering with its function.
- The total DRUJ is a solution to those cases with absence of the sigmoid notch, poor soft tissue, or too much ulnar bone resected.
- The ability of patients to return to regular activities is documented, with 5-year follow-up.

HISTORY AND EVOLUTION OF THE TECHNIQUE

The DRUJ is well known for its contribution to forearm pronation and supination. Less known is its importance for grip strength and lifting capabilities. Two forces act in the forearm: axial loading, which occurs during gripping, and a transverse force, transmitted from the hand to the radius to the ulnar head during lifting.[1] The ulna, acting as the axis of the forearm, supports the radius throughout its range of motion and provides flexion and extension at the elbow. The support provided by the ulna allows the radius to rotate in space as it transfers axial load to the humerus.[2,3]

Mechanical derangement of the distal radioulnar articulation has serious effects on its function. The etiologic spectrum for this derangement can range from early arthritic erosion to the resection of part or all of the distal ulna.[4] Various resections, as described by Darrach, Watson, Bowers, and Sauvé-Kapandji, can lead to a condition known as *ulnar impingement*. This condition occurs because the now unsupported distal end of the radius falls against the adjacent ulnar shaft. At this stage, the term, ulnar impingement, conjures up a picture of an ulna that moves and impinges against the radius, but, in reality, the opposite is true.[5]

Historically, the resections for DRUJ arthritis have been largely successful for pain relief and improved range of motion. Pain persists, however, with gripping and lifting. To address ulnar impingement, ulnar head replacement procedures have been developed. Unfortunately, these may lead to painful erosion of the sigmoid notch due to modular mismatch between the prosthesis and the bone. Unconstrained DRUJ replacements treat the problem with sigmoid notch erosion but they cannot adequately address patients with an unstable distal radioulnar joint. Therefore, the solution for pain relief, range of motion, durability, and stability is the semiconstrained DRUJ arthroplasty.

INDICATIONS FOR THE PROCEDURE

The term, *constraint*, means restriction or limitation. Prostheses that have limitations frequently break or become loose as a result of forces not able to find

Disclosure: One of the authors (LRS) is part owner of Aptis Medical, LLC, manufacturer of the Scheker total DRUJ replacement prosthesis; DWM has nothing to disclose.

[a] Christine M. Kleinert Institute for Hand and Micro Surgery, 225 Abraham Flexner Way #700, Louisville, KY 40202, USA; [b] Division of Plastic and Reconstructive Surgery, University of Louisville, School of Medicine, Louisville, KY 40292, USA; [c] The Core Institute, 2730 East Agua Fria Freeway #100, Phoenix, AZ 85027, USA
* Corresponding author. Christine M. Kleinert Institute for Hand and Micro Surgery, 225 Abraham Flexner Way, #700, Louisville, KY 40202.
E-mail address: lscheker@kleinertkutz.com

a pass-through route due to the limitation in motion. The authors have created an implant that does not have a stop point and restores the function of the joint in its totality, even though the appearance is not that of the normal joint. This device allows full pronation and supination, radial migration, and variable angle of rotation. The prosthesis is indicated for patients with mature skeletons who have rheumatoid, degenerative, or posttraumatic arthritis of the DRUJ and who may or may not have already had surgical treatment. It is especially useful for a failed and painful Darrach procedure, Sauvé-Kapandji procedure, matched resection, or similar types of bone excision or for failed and unstable unipolar ulna head replacement and unconstrained DRUJ arthroplasties. The prosthesis has proved of great use for individuals who need distal ulna resection for tumors and for patients with congenital abnormalities, such as Madelung deformity and Ehlers-Danlos syndrome. Also, in the acute traumatic setting, it may be used for severe fractures of the ulnar head or neck not amenable to good reduction and proper fixation.

Preoperative graded radiographs are used to determine the size of the prosthesis that is required for each case. Elongated ulnar stems can be used in those individuals who have lost large segments of the ulna (more than 5 cm). The device can be used in patients who have at least 11 cm of proximal ulna remaining, allowing the stem to be implanted properly. In general, patients with more ulna length and those in whom the DRUJ replacement is the initial DRUJ procedure have better function.[6]

Contraindications include severe osteoporosis, unresolved osteomyelitis, and systemic disease that debilitate patients both physically and mentally. The use of the implant is also contraindicated when bone, musculature, tendons, or adjacent soft tissues are compromised by disease or infection and would not provide adequate support or fixation for the prosthesis. The implant should not be used in patients who have not reached skeletal maturity.

CURRENT TECHNIQUE

The Aptis DRUJ prosthesis consists of a semiconstrained and modular implant designed to replace the function of the ulnar head, the sigmoid notch of the radius, and the triangular fibrocartilage ligaments. The ulnar components consist of an endomedullary stem made of a cobalt chromium alloy, titanium plasma spray, and an ultra-high-molecular weight (UHMW) polyethylene ball (**Fig. 1**). The plasma spray on the distal third of the ulnar stem promotes bone ingrowth, creating

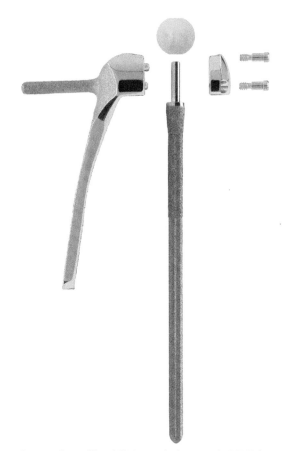

Fig. 1. The self-stabilizing Scheker total DRUJ has a radius plate with a distal socket, an ulnar stem with an UHMW polyethylene ball, and a ball cover to complete the assembly. The advantage is that it does not require any ligaments from the original joint to be available to work.

a stronger fixation through osseointegration. This component of the prosthesis is press-fit inside the ulnar medullary cavity. The radial component provides the socket for the joint and consists of 2 parts that are assembled intraoperatively. The main part is shaped in the form of a plate with a hemisocket on the distal end and a radial peg on the opposite side. The plate is contoured to fit against the distal radius, on its ulnar side, in the area proximal to the sigmoid notch. The plate is fixed to the radius by a peg and 4 or 5 specially designed 3.5-mm cortical screws, depending on the size of the plate. The hemisocket, which is part of the plate, is directed ulnarward and is designed to receive the UHMW polyethylene ball of the ulnar component. The other half of the socket, a cap or cover, is fixed to its counterpart on the plate by means of 2 pegs and 2 small screws. This assembly is accomplished intraoperatively over the UHMW polyethylene ball of the ulna component.

The procedure is generally performed under axillary block. An iodine plastic wrap is used to avoid contact between the implant and the skin. A tourniquet is always applied for improved visualization. An 8-cm longitudinal incision in the shape of a hockey stick is made along the ulnar border of the distal forearm, in the interval between the fifth and sixth dorsal compartments. Care is taken to avoid damage to the sensory branches of the ulnar nerve. The skin and subcutaneous flap are elevated up to the radial wrist extensors. A rectangular ulnar-based fascial flap is created with enough width to cover the head of the implant; it may include the most proximal part of the extensor retinaculum (**Fig. 2**). This flap is be used later to create a buffering barrier between the prosthesis and the extensor carpi ulnaris (ECU).

The dissection is continued between the extensor digiti minimi and the ECU until the ulna is encountered and the extensor digiti minimi is elevated from the ulna and the interosseous membrane for at least 8 cm. The sensory branch of the posterior interosseous nerve is divided to avoid avulsion of the nerve from the thumb extensors when placing an elevator between the extensor mass and the radius. The sheath of the ECU tendon is opened distally up to its insertion at the base of the fifth metacarpal to avoid pressure against the distal end of the implant. The head of the ulna, if present, is then excised at a level just proximal to the cartilage or where the DRUJ would have been (**Fig. 3**).

At this point, the radial attachment of the triangular fibrocartilage, if found intact, is left undisturbed. This structure can provide a barrier between the prosthesis and the carpal bones. The ulnar shaft is then retracted in a palmar direction, thus allowing access to the radius. The interosseous membrane is elevated from the radius along the

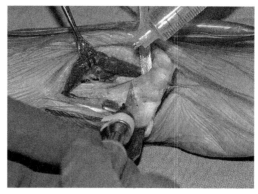

Fig. 3. When the ulnar head is present, the osteotomy is done at the neck of the ulna to allow the trial plate to be placed on the ulnar side of the radius. If the patient had a previous ulnar head excision, and if the plate can be placed in position, the osteotomy is performed in such a way to find a good medullary cavity, which accommodates the required ulnar stem with extended collar.

distal 8 cm of the interosseous crest. The radial trial plate is then placed over the interosseous crest of the radius, and its anterior border is aligned with the anterior surface of the radius. Care is taken to ensure that at least 3 mm of the sigmoid notch lies distal to the end of the plate. Depending on the anatomy encountered, the distal radius may require contouring, including removal of the volar lip of the sigmoid notch with a saw blade or a medium-sized burr ball. After the position of the trial plate has been deemed appropriate—meaning parallel to the anterior shaft of the radius and at least 3 mm proximal to the end of the radius—a 1.4-mm (0.054-in) Kirschner wire is inserted in 1 of the holes at the distal end of the trial component as well as in the most proximal hole (**Fig. 4**).

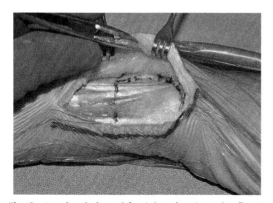

Fig. 2. An ulnarly based fascial and retinacular flap is elevated for use as a buffer between the implant and the ECU. The flap extends radially to the second compartment and is 4 cm in width.

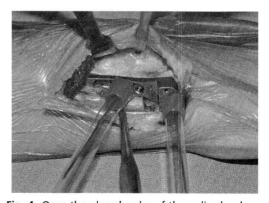

Fig. 4. Once the ulnar border of the radius has been prepared to accommodate the trial plate, 2 Kirschner wires are used to secure the plate against the radius. Image intensifier is used to check placement of the trial plate both in anteroposterior and lateral views.

An image intensifier is used to check the position of the trial, both in anteroposterior and lateral positions. If no adjustment is needed, a 2.5-mm drill bit is used with the provided guide to drill the screw hole at the oval opening of the plate, the proper screw length is measured, the hole is tapped, and the appropriate 3.5-mm screw is inserted. The image intensifier is used again to confirm plate positioning and proper screw length. With confirmation of the length of the screw and good plate contact with the bone, the distal Kirschner wire is removed, and the hole for the radial peg is drilled with appropriate drill bit. When the surgeon is satisfied with the positioning, the trial component is removed and replaced with the prosthesis' radial component. If necessary, a soft mallet is used to achieve good contact between the radius plate and the ulnar border of the radius.

After the last screw is inserted, a final check of the radius plate to confirm screw length and position is performed with the image intensifier. Attention is now turned to the ulna. With the forearm fully pronated, a measuring device with an appropriate color ball (blue for a large implant and black for a small implant) is held into the hemisocket of the radial component. The measuring device is juxtaposed against the ulna shaft. This enables the surgeon to assess the exact amount of ulna to be resected (**Fig. 5**).

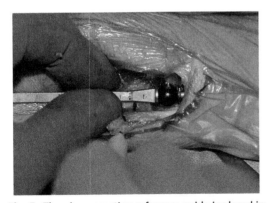

Fig. 5. The ulnar resection reference guide is placed in the socket of the prosthesis to determine the level of osteotomy of the ulna. There are 2 different balls according to the size of the plate—the blue ball is for the 30 plate and the black ball for the 20 plate. It is important that the ball is tightly fixed at the end of the reference guide. After the osteotomy, the reference guide should be again placed into position to check that the osteotomy was performed where intended. If the osteotomy is distal to the desired level, further resection is required; otherwise, the stem will not be inserted to the needed position. If too much is removed, then the stem needs to be inserted only until the end of the highly polished peg is level to the distal end of the plate.

After resection of the distal ulna, a 1.6-mm (0.062-in) guide wire is inserted into the ulna medullary canal to act as a guide for a cannulated drill bit. The canal is drilled for a length of 11 cm. Next, a medullary broach of appropriate size is inserted into the canal to bevel the distal ulna and plane its distal end (**Fig. 6**).

The medullary canal is now thoroughly irrigated, and the stem of the ulnar component is introduced. Next, the UHMW polyethylene ball is placed over the distal peg of the ulnar component and is positioned within the hemisocket of the radial component. Finally, the other half of the radial socket cover is positioned over the ball and secured with 2 small screws. The image intensifier is once again used to confirm adequacy of implant position (**Fig. 7**). Full range of motion is confirmed. The fascia and retinaculum flap are placed between the prosthesis and the ECU tendon and sutured to the radius. This prevents tenosynovitis of the ECU and provides a cushion over the implant, especially for a patient with little subcutaneous adipose tissue. The tourniquet is released, and complete hemostasis is achieved. The skin is then closed with interrupted sutures and a bulky soft dressing is applied.

POSTOPERATIVE PROTOCOL

In the initial publication of 2001, the patients were routinely placed in a long arm splint in neutral position for 3 weeks. After 3 weeks, the splint was removed and active range of motion was encouraged. If needed, physical therapy was initiated at that time. As the authors have gained experience, they have realized that splinting is not necessary. Currently, patients receive a bulky soft dressing and immediate limited motion can begin according to patient tolerance. The dressing remains in

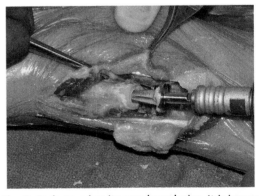

Fig. 6. Each stem has its own broach size. It is important that the broach is introduced until the flare touches the end of the ulna to ensure that the stem will sit at the right level with the head of the plate.

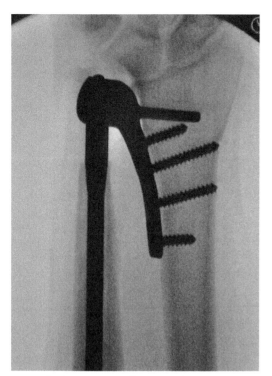

Fig. 7. The image intensifier is used to evaluate the implant position and screw length. At the end of the procedure it is used with the forearm placed through continuous range of motion to verify there is no contact between the end of the ulna and the plate, as could happen with a wide distal ulna.

position for 2 weeks, at which time the sutures are removed and full range-of-motion exercises are encouraged. Therapy is initiated, if necessary, with active range of motion. Without the possibility of dislocation, patients can both move through a full range of motion and bear weight immediately after surgery.

The authors understand that the concept of weight bearing by the head of the ulna is not universally accepted; therefore, this concept needs to be explained. The term, *weight bearing*, has been reserved for the lower extremities, but the vertebrae of the cervical spine each carry the weight of the structures above them, meaning the atlas carries the weight of the head while C7 carries the weight of the head and all the vertebrae above it. Elbow flexion is achieved at all times by the brachialis anterior that inserts distal to the coronoid process of the ulna. The biceps works as a strong elbow flexor after the forearm is fully supinated whereas the brachioradialis is not a voluntary muscle and its work is to modulate elbow extension. When moved from a pure vertical axis, in neutral rotation, the DRUJ is subject to compression imparted by way of the upward force of the ulna and downward force

exerted by gravity acting on the mass of the hand and anything held in the hand. In this way, the DRUJ acts as a weight-bearing joint, bearing a load imparted by mass in the plane of gravitational acceleration. No difference exists when comparing the way that the hip bears the load of gravity on body mass in the standing position (**Fig. 8**).

RESULTS
First-Generation Prosthesis

Between May 1997 and August 2001, 31 patients underwent total DRUJ prosthesis arthroplasty using the initial Scheker prosthesis, made of 316 medical-grade stainless steel and with a 3-point fixation of the 3-mm ulnar stem.[7] At long-term follow-up (mean 5.9 years, range 4–8 years), all 31 patients scored a mean patient-rated wrist evaluation (PRWE) of 29 (range 1–68) after implantation of the DRUJ prosthesis, and the mean disabilities of the arm, shoulder and hand (DASH) score was 23 (range 0–76). Subjectively, these 31 patients scored preoperative pain on a 5-point scale at a mean of 4.2 (range 1–5) and postoperative pain at 1.0 (range 0–4). Mean pronation was 79° (range 15–90°) and mean supination was 72° (range 30–90°) at final follow-up. In the 22 wrists that had not previously undergone partial or total wrist fusion, mean extension was 56° (range 14–90°) and mean flexion was 52° (range 5–85°) at final follow-up. Mean ulnar deviation was 21.5° (range 5–30°) and mean radial deviation was 10.5° (range 5–15°) at final follow-up.

Preoperatively, grip strength was a mean of 25 lb (range 0–80 lb); postoperatively, it was a mean of 49 lb (range 0–100 lb) for the operated side, compared with an average of 80 lb (range 20–114 lb) for the contralateral side. Twenty-nine patients were able to bear weight on the operative side (range 5–20 lb); 13 of these were able to lift 10 lb or more, 11 without any pain in the neutral position. Eight were able to lift 20 lb, 5 without any pain in the neutral position. Lifting in the pronated position, these patients were able to bear a mean weight of 15 lb (range 5–20 lb) but experienced pain at approximately half the weight lifted in the neutral position. Two patients with reflex sympathetic dystrophy had reduced grip strength both preoperatively and postoperatively and were unable to bear weight.

Twenty-four of the 31 patients returned to their regular activities, 4 returned to their previous activities with a permanent weight-bearing restriction, 1 patient filed for disability, and 2 patients retired. The 2 patients who retired stated that they had no problems with their activities of daily living. The youngest patient, aged 18, completed studies to become a small animal veterinarian and has continued in this activity without problems. No implant has

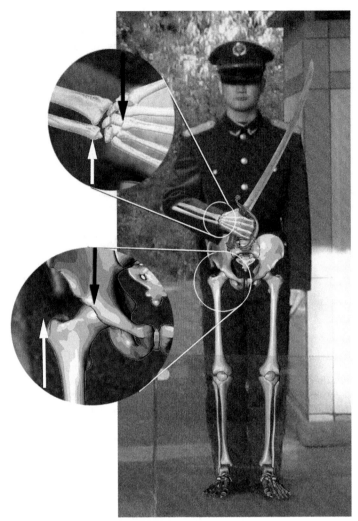

Fig. 8. The weight of the sword is carried by the head of the ulna in the same way that the weight of the right side of the body is carried by the head of the femur. The black arrows show the force of gravity acting on the head of the femur and the head of the ulna. The white arrows depict the forces fighting gravity to maintain position.

been reported to have failed under normal conditions. At final follow-up radiograph, all 31 cases demonstrated no radiolucency around the implant.

Second-Generation Prosthesis

The original prosthesis was changed from medical-grade 316 stainless steel to cobalt chromium with a titanium plasma spray. This prosthesis was cleared for regular use by the Food and Drug Administration in January 2005. Since the pilot study was finished and published in 2009,[8] from 2005 onward the senior author (LRS) has successfully treated more than 231 patients with deranged DRUJs. A 5-year follow-up study was conducted of the first 35 patients treated with the Food and Drug Administration–cleared prosthesis to evaluate the results. Data showed significant improvement in

all categories of patient function. Mean range of motion increased to normative ranges at 5 years, increasing pronation from 62° to 83° and supination from 51° to 75°. Grip strength increased from an average 31 lb to 51 lb, or from 44% to 94%, of the contralateral side. Pain decreased significantly, both at rest and with activity.

At 5-year follow-up, forearm weight bearing in neutral position was an average 16.3 pounds in the DRUJ prosthesis arm versus 16.8 pounds in the contralateral upper extremity. There was no significant difference between the lifting capacities of the prosthesis arm versus the opposite arm in either the neutral, pronated, or supinated lifting positions.

Patients expressed an average satisfaction of 9.6 of 10 (10 = completely satisfied) with their prostheses. Five-year postoperative mean DASH score was 14 of 100 (n = 19), and mean PRWE score was

22 of 100 (n = 18). Preoperative DASH and PRWE scores were not available. These postoperative results indicate, however, that patients had minimal pain and difficulty with activities of daily living.

Five-year follow-up postoperative data were obtained in 27 of the first 35 patients to receive the second-generation prosthesis. Among these 27 patients, there was a 100% survival rate of the prosthesis at 5 years. Two minor soft tissue infections occurred during the immediate postoperative period and resolved with antibiotics. There was no evidence of periprosthetic infection on radiographs. Thirty-six prostheses (69%) were complication-free. Eleven (31%) of the prostheses had 12 complications: the authors observed 6 cases of ECU tendonitis, 5 cases of ectopic bone formation, and 1 screw/cap loosening. All complications were resolved surgically with good clinical course and patient satisfaction. One patient suffered from ECU hypersensitivity 4 years postimplant, which was attributed to failed tendon repair before receiving the prosthesis. Nevertheless, her issue was resolved with steroid injection. One patient had his ulnar stem replaced 4 years postoperatively when a larger ulnar stem became available; his original 2005 implant stem was too small for his medullary cavity but the patient, at that time, had elected to receive the prosthesis anyway.

Radiographs of 23 DRUJ prostheses were available at long-term follow-up (mean 5 years, range 4.4–6.2 years postoperatively) for review. Follow-up radiographs were compared with images obtained after the 2005 prosthesis implantations. In 20 prostheses, the authors observed bone regrowth in former screw holes and/or around screws. Bone growth was observed on the proximal edge of the radial plate in 19 cases. Twenty-one prostheses showed no signs of loosening. Two prostheses showed slight evidence of stem loosening, which was asymptomatic for both patients. One prosthesis, in addition to the potential stem loosening, had asymptomatic loosening of a screw on the prosthesis cap as well as ectopic bone growth over approximately one-third of the proximal part of the radial plate. Nevertheless, the patient had no symptoms, reported no pain, and reported utmost satisfaction with his prosthesis. One patient had ectopic bone growth at the top of the ulnar stem, and one patient who underwent stem replacement at 4 years postoperatively showed signs of shock around the screws and radial peg, attributed to his previously placed ulnar stem that was too narrow. The authors replaced the ulnar stem with a 6-mm diameter stem, which has since been added to the armamentarium. Neither of these patients had symptoms, and both reported

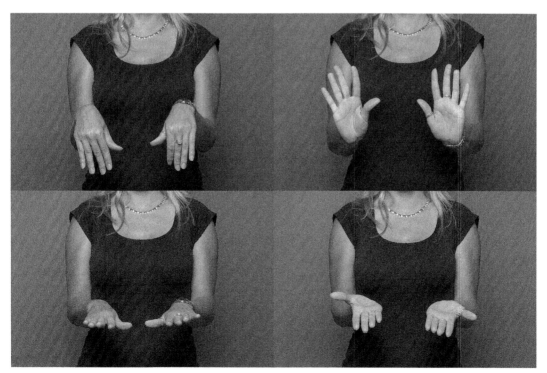

Fig. 9. The prosthesis allows the patient to return to painless motion in pronation and supination without affecting flexion and extension of the wrist (if present before surgery).

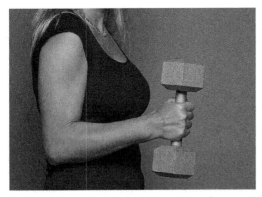

Fig. 10. Patients are able to lift weight without pain. The recommended lifting limit is 20 lb. This is one-seventh of the average strength of the highly polished peg at the end of the stem, as tested by the Instron machine, in which the prostheses were tested to failure. Peg strength varied from 148 to 186 pounds, with an average of 169 lb.

minimal pain and utmost satisfaction with their prostheses.

It has been shown that excision of the head of the ulna leads to impingement and pain with pronation/supination and lifting.[5] Most of these patients have had between 2 and 14 procedures on the DRUJ—from partial excision of the DRUJ to wide excision of the ulna, and all the techniques of soft tissue

stabilization available. Once the total replacement was done, patients were able to use their hand and forearm without limitations, stop taking prescription pain medications, and return to a productive life. Excellent range of motion is achieved (**Fig. 9**). Lifting capacity, which is not possible with salvage procedures, is restored in these patients (**Fig. 10**). More than 200 surgeons worldwide have had experience with the second-generation prosthesis with results similar to ours.

COMPLICATIONS AND HOW TO DEAL WITH THEM

As is the case for any implant arthroplasty, one of the major concerns is postoperative infection. For patients with a low-degree soft tissue infection, antibiotics alone have proved sufficient treatment. These patients often have had multiple previous operations. Deep infection should be treated like any other prosthetic joint replacement with a 2-stage revision arthroplasty. The first stage requires removal of the prosthesis and placement of an antibiotic spacer. Removal can be difficult if the prosthesis is well fixed and may necessitate an osteotomy of the distal ulna. After 6 weeks of antibiotics, removal of the antibiotic spacer and revision arthroplasty is performed. This may require a custom prosthesis depending on the amount of

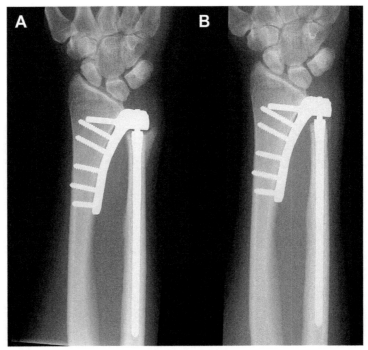

Fig. 11. Radiographs of patient in **Figs. 9** and **10**. (*A*) Ectopic bone formation around the distal end of the ulna causing painful ECU tendinitis. (*B*) Postoperative radiograph with ectopic bone trimmed out.

bone loss due to infection and surgical resection. The implant can be safely inserted as long as at least 11 cm of proximal ulna remains.

Other complications include ECU tenosynovitis, which can be successfully treated (or, preferably, avoided) by creating a fascial flap interposed between the implant and the ECU tendon. Motor vehicle accidents caused the ulnar stems to break in 2 cases of the pilot study. In both cases, the stems were 3 mm in diameter and made of previously used 316 stainless steel, which has since been replaced with cobalt chromium. The prostheses were replaced and the patients regained function and continue unremarkably. Of patients with the new prosthesis, 2 had ectopic bone formation around the distal ulna causing ECU tendinitis and were treated successfully with surgical excision (**Fig. 11**). Both cases were in patients with Madelung deformity. This ectopic calcification was caused by the periosteum not being resected because the head of the ulna was excised in a subperiosteal manner; this can be avoided. Another patient, on the 1-year follow-up radiograph, had some ulna resorption in the distal segment of the ulna where she had an ulnar shortening 6 months before the replacement arthroplasty. At present, the ulnar stem remains well secured and she is symptom-free.

REFERENCES

1. Scheker L, Babb B, Killion P. Distal ulnar prosthetic replacement. Orthop Clin North Am 2001;30:365–76.
2. Hagert CG. The distal radioulnar joint. Hand Clin 1987;3:41–50.
3. Hagert CG. The distal radioulnar joint in relation to the whole forearm [review]. Clin Orthop 1992;275:56–64.
4. Bieber EJ, Linscheid RL, Dobyns JH, et al. Failed distal ulna resections. J Hand Surg 1988;13:193–200.
5. Lees VC, Scheker LR. The radiological demonstration of dynamic ulnar impingement. J Hand Surg Br 1997;22:448–50.
6. Scheker L. Implant arthroplasty for the distal radioulnar joint. J Hand Surg Am 2008;33:1639–44.
7. Laurentin-Pérez L, Goodwin A, Babb B, et al. A study of functional outcomes following implantation of a total distal radioulnar joint prosthesis. J Hand Surg Eur Vol 2008;13:18–28.
8. Scheker L. Arthritis of the distal radioulnar joint. Tech In Ortho 2009;24:32–41.

Rehabilitation Following Thumb CMC, Radiocarpal, and DRUJ Arthroplasty

Carla A. Crosby, PT, CHT*, Jennifer L. Reitz, OTR/L, CHT,
Elizabeth A. Mester, MS, OTR/L, CHT,
Marie-Lyne Grenier, MSc, OTR/L

KEYWORDS

- Rehabilitation • Hand therapy • Arthroplasty • Wrist • CMC joint • DRUJ • Assessment • DJD

KEY POINTS

- Hand therapy is essential after arthroplasty around the wrist.
- This article includes therapy guidelines and goals after surgical reconstruction of the thumb carpometacarpal joint, radiocarpal joint, and distal radioulnar joint.
- Tables and figures are included to guide the hand therapist in the process of returning this patient population to pain-free function.

INTRODUCTION

Arthroplasty surgery of the thumb, wrist, and forearm is always a salvage procedure. These patients desire surgery because the pain and function in their affected extremity is limiting their daily lives. This chapter gives a basic background of each surgery followed by detailed interventions for the hand therapist to incorporate throughout the process of a patient's recovery. Pain-free functional motion with adequate strength is the main goal of all joint reconstructions. Loosening of the prosthesis is a leading cause of poor outcome in arthroplasty. This is usually attributed to mechanical failure, prosthetic fracture, prosthetic malposition, soft tissue imbalance, or excessive joint laxity caused by progression of the arthritic disease process or excessive activity following surgery.[1–8] To protect the prosthesis, patients are discouraged from lifting more than 2 lb regularly and no more than 10 lb

occasionally. Patients should avoid repetitive activities, impact sports, and weight bearing (such as on a cane or crutch) on the involved side.[1,9–11] Patients are encouraged to attend yearly follow-up visits with their surgeon to monitor continued viability and alignment of the prosthesis. Although a significant amount of information regarding postoperative management of arthroplasty exists, no protocols have been subjected to scientific analysis.[12] Current protocols should be used only as a guideline for therapy. They are useful in providing a blueprint for the overall concerns and goals of a particular arthroplasty. Variations are expected because each patient presents differently. Further research is required to determine which therapy guidelines yield the best and most reliable results. This is especially important because therapists must increasingly justify their treatments and worth to insurance companies, managed care organizations, and patients.[11,12] To minimize poor outcome, there is

Disclosure: Authors have nothing to disclose.
Hand Therapy Department, Pennsylvania Hand Center, Bryn Mawr, PA, USA
* Corresponding author. Pennsylvania Hand Center, 101 South Bryn Mawr Avenue, Suite 300, Bryn Mawr, PA 19010.
E-mail address: BMTherapy@pahandcenter.com

a need to gradually increase motion and strength while managing adhesions, joint instability, soft tissue imbalance, implant loosening, and infection.[1] Proper early management of arthroplasty, through planning and awareness of complications, can yield functional pain-free results.

GENERAL ARTHROPLASTY POSTOPERATIVE CARE

After arthroplasty surgery the patient is typically wrapped in a bulky dressing in the operating room. Hand therapy begins 3 to 5 days postoperatively for edema control, protected range of motion (ROM), and wound care. The initial therapy evaluation includes assessment of pain, edema, function, sensation, and upper extremity motion. Pain is assessed by a visual or numerical analog scale. Edema is measured circumferentially or by volume. Sensation is assessed by patient report of symptoms and Semmes-Weinstein monofilaments. Function is evaluated by assessment questionnaires and ROM by goniometric measurements. The patient is initially instructed in a home program including pain control measures, edema control, ROM of the uninvolved joints, splint care, and activities of daily living (ADL) modification to avoid lifting and gripping activities with the operated hand. Pain may be controlled with medication prescribed by the surgeon and use of transcutaneous electric nerve stimulation or interferential nerve stimulation. Edema control includes the use of ice; massage; elevation; and compression garments, such as edema gloves or compression sleeves for use under the protective splint especially while sleeping. Passive ROM (PROM) of the digits is also performed to decrease joint stiffness and prevent adhesions of the dorsal extensors and retinaculum.[1,13] Tendon gliding exercises (TGE) give the patient full excursion of the flexor and extensor tendons in the hand and across the wrist joint.[14] Encouraging the patient to move the elbow, shoulder, and digits decreases upper extremity stiffness; minimizes muscle guarding and overall weakness; and improves circulation, edema, and pain. Patient education is the key to a successful rehabilitation program. The home program should be written out and include details, frequency and duration of each therapeutic intervention, and diagrams or photographs to further instruct the patient. For example, "TGE: 10 repetitions each, three to four times per day" and "retrograde massage: 10 min session, two times per day" improve patient understanding while providing the therapist with information on the effective dose of each intervention. A well-informed patient usually demonstrates good compliance with the rehabilitation program. The patient should be well-versed in exercises, healing timelines, activity restrictions, and expected therapeutic outcomes. For the best possible results, the home program is updated often and its importance emphasized to the patient each time it is reviewed.

Sutures are removed 10 to 14 days postoperatively. Desensitization and the use of an elastomere or silicone pressure pad may begin 3 to 5 days after suture removal. Scar massage starts at 3 weeks postoperatively. To reduce adhesions, phonophoresis may begin 3 to 4 weeks postoperatively just before and throughout the peak of scar formation.[15]

Functional outcome questionnaires, such as the Disabilities of the Arm, Shoulder, and Hand Score (DASH or Quick-DASH)[16] and the Patient Rated Wrist Evaluation,[17] help assess functional progress and can be completed at various intervals during rehabilitation.[18] Functional outcome measurements should be administered preoperatively, at the initial postoperative visit, then monthly, and at the final visit. These assessments identify areas of ability and disability allowing the therapist to establish and achieve specific short and long-term patient goals.[18] A preoperative evaluation including a functional outcome assessment can serve as a baseline to compare future functional measurements, patient satisfaction, and overall improvement after surgery. Postoperative monthly evaluations determine future treatment needs. A final evaluation and follow-up visits reflect the accomplished results. When the arthroplasty is deemed stable and secure enough to start motion of the involved joint, ROM measurements are assessed with a goniometer.

ROM ASSESSMENT
Thumb Carpometacarpal

To measure thumb carpometacarpal (CMC) flexion, the patient is instructed to oppose their thumb and touch the tip of the most ulnar finger they are able to reach comfortably. The patient then slides the thumb down that finger proximally as far as possible without pain. The finger and level touched by the thumb is recorded. Full motion of thumb CMC flexion is across the palm to the fifth metacarpal head and can be abbreviated as "H5" (**Fig. 1**). CMC extension and abduction are measured according to The American Society of Hand Therapists (ASHT) 1992 Clinical Assessment Recommendations. Thumb extension takes place in the plane of the palm (**Fig. 2**) and thumb abduction in a plane at a right angle to the palm (**Fig. 3**). For these motions the goniometer's stationary arm is aligned with the

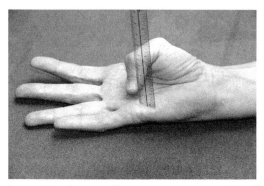

Fig. 1. Thumb CMC flexion ROM. Measured with goniometer from thumb pulp to distal palmar crease overlying the head of the fifth metacarpal; if full, abbreviated "H5" for its ability to reach the head of the fifth metacarpal (Copyright Pennsylvania Hand Center, with permission).

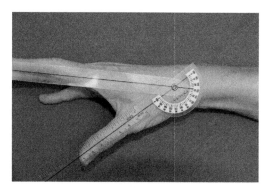

Fig. 3. Thumb CMC abduction ROM measurement with goniometer (Copyright Pennsylvania Hand Center, with permission).

second metacarpal, and the movable arm is aligned with the first metacarpal.[19]

Wrist

Wrist ROM measurements are best taken from the ulnar side of the wrist. ASHT recommends measuring wrist motion from the dorsal or radial aspect of the wrist.[19] This method, however, is impractical because swelling often interferes with the goniometer's dorsal placement on the wrist and the thumb interferes with radial placement of the goniometer. Wrist ROM measurements are best taken from the ulnar side of the wrist (**Fig. 4**). The stationary arm of the goniometer is placed on the ulnar side of the forearm, the joint axis is aligned with the joint of the prosthesis, and the movable arm of the goniometer is aligned with the third metacarpal. With practice, visualizing the joint axis through skin provides for an accurate measurement. This method of "seeing through the soft

tissue," as if with x-ray vision, is helpful when measuring edematous or deformed joints (**Fig. 5**).

Forearm

As described in the ASHT's recommendations, forearm rotation is best measured with the involved arm at the patient's side, the elbow flexed to 90 degrees, and the forearm in neutral with the thumb pointing toward the ceiling.[20] This neutral forearm position is the starting point and measured as "zero" for pronation and supination. The goniometer's stationary arm is aligned vertically with the patient's arm (**Figs. 6** and **7**). To measure supination, the patient rotates the forearm to the maximum palm-up position with the goniometer's movable arm parallel to and resting on the flexion crease at the wrist flexion crease (**Fig. 6**). To measure pronation, the patient rotates the forearm to the maximum palm-down position with the goniometer's movable arm parallel to and resting on the dorsal or palmar aspect of the wrist, or in the palm (**Fig. 7**). In both directions, the axis of the goniometer is placed at the ulnar styloid. Once again,

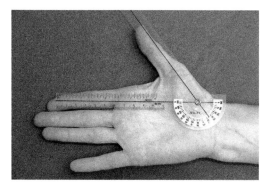

Fig. 2. Thumb CMC extension ROM measurement with goniometer (Copyright Pennsylvania Hand Center, with permission).

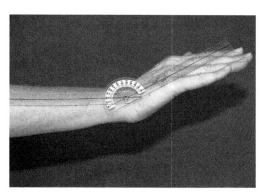

Fig. 4. Wrist extension and flexion ROM measured with goniometer from ulnar side. (Copyright Pennsylvania Hand Center, with permission).

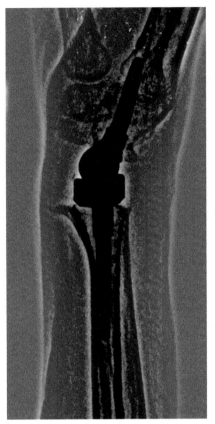

Fig. 5. "X-ray vision" at wrist. Visualizing the joint and bone structure through the soft tissue is important. This radiograph shows 30 degrees of actual wrist extension, whereas the outside skin appearance only reveals 5 degrees of extension (Copyright Pennsylvania Hand Center, with permission).

a therapist's "x-ray vision" of the bony anatomy is necessary to visualize the distal radioulnar joint (DRUJ) as the radius rotates over the ulna. In the uninjured population, full supination is approximately 90 degrees, whereas pronation is approximately 80 degrees.[21] Recent analysis of forearm position during functional tasks identified the degrees of pronation and supination required to perform modern daily tasks in 25 subjects.[22] Opening a door required 77 degrees of supination while typing on a keyboard required 65 degrees of pronation. For various contemporary tasks, the minimum supination necessary was 65 degrees, whereas minimum pronation needed was 60 degrees.

THERAPY AFTER THUMB CMC ARTHROPLASTY

Trapeziometacarpal arthritis is commonly referred to as thumb CMC or basal joint arthritis. Pantrapezial arthritis refers to the additional involvement of the scaphotrapezial joint. The scaphotrapezoid joint is also involved frequently. These conditions are associated with pain at the base of the thumb causing difficulty in hand function. The basal joint is susceptible to breakdown because of high compressive forces of up to 26 lbs with pinch and lbs with strong grip.[23] Arthritis of the thumb CMC joint is associated with decreased motion, especially abduction and extension.[24] Activities requiring lateral pinch or a wide grip are often the most painful.[25] This also limits the ability to release, grip, or push large objects.[24] Achieving full CMC extension is usually the most difficult goal. This is necessary for full breadth of grip, improved strength, and better cosmetic appeal.

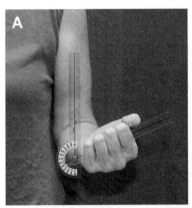
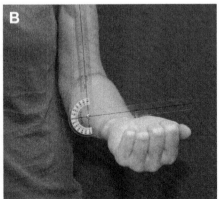

Fig. 6. Forearm supination measurement techniques with a goniometer can vary. Consistent alignment of the goniometer's arms with the humerus and distal forearm is an important factor. The forearm limb of the goniometer can be placed in the palm (*A*) or at the wrist flexion crease (*B*) (Copyright Pennsylvania Hand Center, with permission).

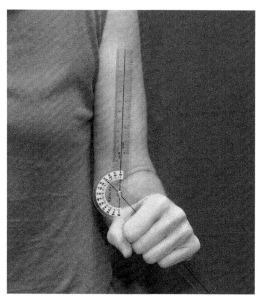

Fig. 7. Forearm pronation ROM measurement with a goniometer. Consistent placement of the goniometer limbs is again important for reproducible readings (Copyright Pennsylvania Hand Center, with permission).

Limited CMC extension can lead to a thumb swan neck deformity. A swan neck deformity is a zigzag deformity caused by ligament laxity resulting in CMC joint flexion, metacarpophalangeal (MP) joint hyperextension, and interphalangeal (IP) joint flexion (**Fig. 8**).[26,27] If the first metacarpal collapses in flexion, the loss of CMC extension limits grip and release of objects.

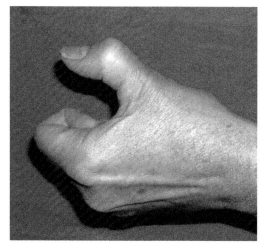

Fig. 8. Swan neck deformity of thumb. Notice compensatory hyperextension at MP joint, secondary to the adduction contracture at the CMC joint (Copyright Pennsylvania Hand Center, with permission).

Women are more likely than men to have trapeziometacarpal arthritis, and both genders have increased risk with age.[28,29] A 2006 radiographic study found that 21% of women compared with 17.7% of men age 40 years or older demonstrate radiographic evidence of thumb CMC osteoarthritis.[28] Another study found a 40% prevalence of thumb CMC degenerative joint disease in women older than 75 years.[29] The primary reasons people seek medical attention for this disorder are pain, weak pinch and grip, and enlargement at the base of the first metacarpal.[25] When pain becomes disabling and hand function is severely affected despite conservative management, arthroplasty is indicated.

Thumb arthroplasties have many variations. Usually, if there are many types of surgeries for a specific problem, it indicates that none is perfect, and even the most advanced solutions have limitations. Procedure selection depends on the severity and specifics found during clinical examination and on radiographs, as well as surgeon preference. Because the basal joint involves multiple carpal bones and articular surfaces, each case is unique. Surgery can include full or partial removal of the trapezium with or without the trapezoid and with or without a tendon interposition, spacer, or prosthesis.

Proximal migration of the first metacarpal is possible after total removal of the trapezium. Over time, this migration causes a shortening of the thumb's length and impingement between the base of the metacarpal and scaphoid.[30–32] Suspension with a Mersilene sling has recently been developed to prevent the first metacarpal from migrating proximally. This procedure provides enough stability to allow for immediate active ROM (AROM) of the reconstructed joint. Less time is needed immobilizing the first CMC with this method than is needed after traditional trapezium resection arthroplasties. Irrespective of which procedure is chosen, the final goal of all arthroplasty surgery is a pain-free stable joint with improved mobility and functional strength. Trapezium resection arthroplasty with Mersilene sling suspension (MSS) and trapezium resection arthroplasty with flexor carpi radialis (FCR) tendon interposition are the procedures of choice at the Pennsylvania Hand Center.

Postoperative Management of Trapezium Resection Arthroplasty with MSS

Immediately postoperative
In the first postoperative visit, the patient is fitted with a protective forearm-based thermoplastic thumb spica splint holding the wrist neutral, the thumb in maximal available CMC extension, and

the MP in 10 degrees of flexion with IP free (**Fig. 9** and **Table 1**). The splint is worn full-time except during exercises and hygiene. As thumb CMC extension improves, the splint is adjusted to further increase CMC extension. The goal is to obtain full thumb CMC extension by 12 weeks postoperatively. This improves grip and prevents CMC subluxation. MP flexion should be encouraged because patients with a previous thumb swan neck deformity have a tendency to settle with MP hyperextension and CMC flexion. A slight flexion contracture at the thumb MP joint allows for more extension at the CMC joint improving overall hand function. This is true even if a trigger-thumb release is performed at the same time as the trapezium arthroplasty.

Two to 4 weeks postoperative

AROM is introduced without restrictions and usually done three to four times per day, 10 repetitions each. This may include TGEs and additional thumb AROM, such as CMC flexion, extension, abduction, adduction, opposition, circumduction, retropulsion, and MP and IP flexion and extension. ADLs including joint protection, body mechanics, and ergonomic education are periodically reviewed with the patient and depend on patient progress, ability, and lifestyle.

Often with thumb arthroplasties, the wrist becomes stiff in flexion and extension. Early attention to wrist ROM can prevent this from occurring. At 4 weeks postoperatively, PROM of the wrist and CMC joint is initiated. To improve wrist motion, a jug filled with 1 to 2 lb of water can be gripped loosely, forcing the wrist to flex or extend over the edge of a table (**Fig. 10**). Allow a stretch of 2 minutes in each direction. Additional pressure with the uninvolved hand can also help promote wrist mobility (**Fig. 11**). A variety of exercises with easily found

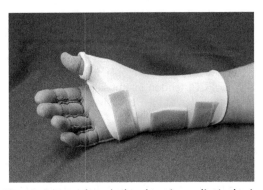

Fig. 9. Forearm-based thumb spica splint/orthosis. Wrist neutral, first CMC in extension, and thumb IP free. (Copyright Pennsylvania Hand Center, with permission).

equipment may also be used for wrist stretching, such as a table-top, chair, or wall push-ups (**Fig. 12**).

Four to 12 weeks postoperative

At 4 weeks postoperatively the thermoplastic splint is reduced to heavy activity only and night time. The patient is offered a neoprene CMC splint for support during the day for mild activities (**Fig. 13**). At 6 weeks postoperatively the thermoplastic splint is discontinued and the neoprene splint is used as needed. Light strengthening of forearm muscles and grip strength begin at 4 weeks postoperatively. Strengthening is gradually increased until the patient is discharged from therapy. Aggressive strengthening is avoided. Thumb CMC extension is difficult for these patients to achieve, and special attention is often needed to gain full extension of the reconstructed CMC joint. A static progressive splint may be required (**Fig. 14**). This splint is fabricated from hard thermoplastic material. The pattern is an ulnar-sided forearm gutter with a dorsoradial flare that is rolled onto itself to create a 1- to 2-in high bridge. A cuff is fabricated out of 2-in neoloop, plain Velcro, or stiff vinyl-leather. To pull the CMC joint into extension, the cuff is placed under the first metacarpal proximal to the thumb MP joint. A practice sling may be used, with a crochet hook, to evaluate the correct line of pull before marking the splint (**Fig. 15**). The cuff is pulled with Velcro over the bridge and attached to the proximal ulnar side of the splint. The patient can gradually self-adjust the force of CMC extension. A thin piece of Velcro attached palmarly between the cuff and the splint can anchor the cuff, to prevent it from slipping distally and extending the MP joint instead of the CMC joint. The splint is worn 1 hour before bedtime and the extension force is gradually increased to full tolerance. The patient is then instructed to loosen the cuff slightly for sleep. This primes the joint and minimizes discomfort while sleeping with the splint. If the patient is unable to wear the splint to bed, it can be worn at intervals throughout the day. To achieve CMC extension with a low-load prolonged stretch, wear time should be approximately 1 to 2 hours, two to four times per day. Therapy is continued until the patient gains full thumb opposition, extension, functional hand strength, and the scar is soft and nontender.

Postoperative Management of Ligament Reconstruction and Tendon Interposition Arthroplasty

Immediately postoperative

Ligament reconstruction with tendon interposition arthroplasty techniques varies (**Table 2**). Generally,

Table 1
Thumb CMC arthroplasty with mersilene sling suspension: therapy guidelines

Postoperative	Immediately	3–5 D	4 Wk	6 Wk	6–8 Wk	8–12 Wk
Splint	Bulky postoperative dressing applied.	Forearm-based thumb spica with CMC in extension, MP slight flexion, and IP free. Worn FT except hygiene and controlled AROM.	Splint decreased to night use and ADLs only. Splint adjusted to maximize thumb CMC extension. A neoprene CMC splint may be used for light ADLs instead of the hard splint.	Patient increases ADLs out of splint. Neoprene splint is used as needed with activity.	Static-progressive thumb CMC extension splint if needed.	Neoprene splint as needed with activity.
Therapy	Pain and edema control. AROM of uninvolved joints.	Pain and edema control. Wound care. AROM and AAROM of thumb, fingers, and wrist. Sutures removed postoperative Day 10.	Continue pain and edema control. AROM and AAROM of thumb, fingers, and wrist. Light resistive strengthening for forearm and grip. Begin scar control.	Continue scar control and light resistive exercises. Continue thumb, finger, and wrist AROM. Start PROM to increase CMC extension.	Continue AROM exercises. Increase resistive exercises but avoid aggressive pinch. Focus on functional strength.	Return to regular activities.
Examples	Ice, elevation, TENS, TGEs, AROM of uninvolved joints.	Wrist and thumb AROM. TGE's. Jobst pump, retrograde massage, and compression gloves for edema. TENS and ice for pain control as needed.	Continue exercise with focus on thumb CMC extension. Start ultrasound or phonophoresis to surgical scars, scar massage, and scar pads.	BTE, Thera-Putty and functional tasks to increase AROM and strength.	Progress strengthening as tolerated. Increase use during ADLs.	Return to ADLs and hobbies pain-free.
Precautions	Monitor for signs of infection and tight dressings.	Monitor for splint fit, nerve compressions, and signs of infection.	Monitor for signs of overuse of thumb, such as increased pain and edema. Encourage splint use to limit activity, if necessary.	Monitor for scar thickening and adhesions. Monitor for signs of overuse of thumb; adjust exercises and splint use accordingly.	Monitor for scar thickening and overuse.	Monitor overuse with activity.

Abbreviations: AAROM, active assisted range of motion; ADLs, activities of daily living; AROM, active range of motion; BTE, Baltimore Therapeutic Equipment; FT, full time; PROM, passive range of motion; ROM, range of motion; TENS, transcutaneous electrical nerve stimulation; TGE, tendon gliding exercises.

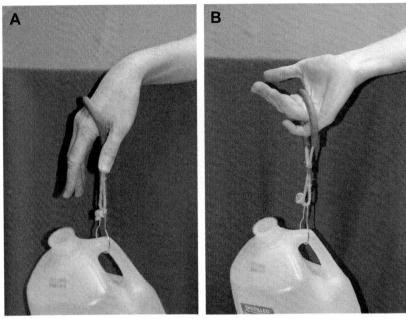

Fig. 10. Jug stretch for wrist flexion (*A*) and extension (*B*). Cord threaded through a rubber tube with a "stopper" bead to adjust around the patient's hand. A curtain hook attaches to the handle of a water jug filled with a tolerable amount of water (Copyright Pennsylvania Hand Center, with permission).

the trapezium is excised, a hole is drilled through the base of the first metacarpal, and a portion of the FCR tendon is passed through the hole. A portion of the FCR is rolled into an "anchovy" and placed into the trapezium space.[31] After this procedure, the patient is immobilized in a cast for 4 to 6 weeks.[25,33] During this phase, hand therapy is limited to edema control, ROM of the uninvolved joints, ADL education, and preventing any nerve compression. Healing time and the rehabilitation program are also reviewed with the patient.

Four to 6 weeks postoperative
Rehabilitation at this point is similar to the MSS protocol. When the cast is removed, the patient is fitted with a thermoplastic thumb spica splint to wear full-time except for ROM exercises and hygiene. The splint is fitted with the wrist in neutral,

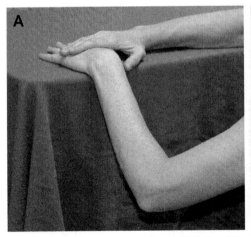
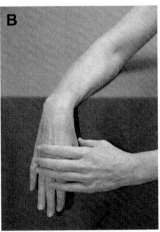

Fig. 11. Wrist stretching exercises at table edge, with help of the opposite hand. Body weight can be brought to bear on the wrist, through the arm (*A*), or just hand force is applied to the stiff wrist (*B*) (Copyright Pennsylvania Hand Center, with permission).

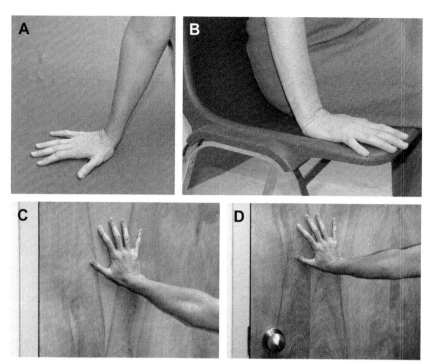

Fig. 12. Wrist stretching pushups: with table top (*A*) or chair (*B*). Wall push-ups: high hand placement (*C*) for gentle extension stretch, lower hand placement (*D*) for more vigorous extension stretch (Copyright Pennsylvania Hand Center, with permission).

thumb CMC in extension, MP in slight flexion, and IP free (**Fig. 9**). Patients may begin light ADLs while wearing the splint. The focus of therapy in this phase is active and active-assisted CMC abduction and extension while avoiding CMC flexion and adduction. Full CMC flexion to the base of the fifth digit is avoided until the thumb can oppose each digit with ease. This prevents stress on the healing ligaments.[25,33] Exercises include thumb IP and MP joint flexion and extension with the first

metacarpal supported in extension by the patient's other hand. Full wrist and finger ROM is encouraged.

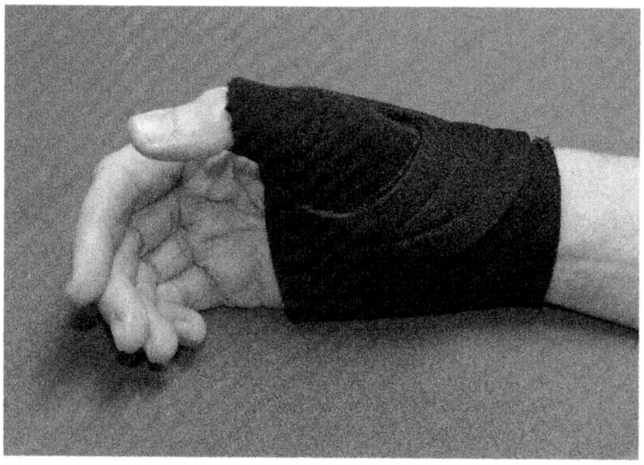

Six to 12 weeks postoperative

At 6 weeks postoperatively the patient can do light functional activities out of the splint and start low-resistance exercises for strength. At 8 weeks, the patient is weaned from the protective splint and increased pinch and grip exercises are encouraged. The static-progressive splint may be needed to achieve full CMC extension (**Fig. 14**). Functional use of the thumb is gradually increased and unrestricted by 12 weeks postoperatively.[25]

Special Considerations

Occasionally, surgery includes a release of the first dorsal compartment, trigger thumb, or carpal tunnel, or an MP arthrodesis or capsulodesis. If MP hyperextension is greater than 30 degrees, MP joint arthrodesis is considered with the CMC reconstruction.[25] Pins may be inserted across the MP joint to prevent motion and may remain in place for many weeks. Therapy must address all surgical procedures accompanying the arthroplasty. After the immobilization phase, AROM is extremely important to regain tendon gliding and reduce adhesions. The patient may also require arthritis

Fig. 13. Neoprene CMC support. Provides wrist and thumb support while allowing some joint motion (Copyright Pennsylvania Hand Center, with permission).

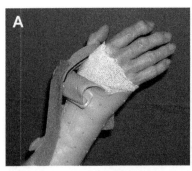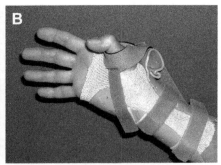

Fig. 14. Thumb CMC static-progressive extension splint/orthosis. Forearm ulnar gutter with "bridge" for proper alignment of thumb CMC Velcro cuff. Dorsal view (*A*) and palmar view (*B*) (Copyright Pennsylvania Hand Center, with permission).

education due to multiple joint degeneration and nerve protection, because joint breakdown often accompanies nerve compression symptoms.

THERAPY AFTER WRIST ARTHROPLASTY

Radiocarpal joint reconstruction, commonly referred to as wrist arthroplasty, is reserved for individuals who seek medical attention because severe and progressive wrist pain limits their activities. These patients present with joint deterioration on radiographs, which may be the result of chronic rheumatoid arthritis, osteoarthritis, or a past traumatic injury. Often symptoms are bilateral and previous interventions have failed. Wrist arthroplasty is carefully considered and preferred over wrist arthrodesis in patients with good bone quality. The lifestyle of these patients should be relatively sedentary because greater dexterity rather than strength is accomplished.[1,4]

Wrist motion needed for everyday activities has been documented most notably in two studies. In

the study by Palmer et al.[34] of 10 subjects, the wrist required 30 degrees of extension, 5 degrees of flexion, 10 degrees of radial deviation, and 15 degrees of ulnar deviation to complete the functional tasks examined. In the study by Ryu et al.[35] of 20 men and 20 women, the requirement was 60 degrees of wrist extension, 54 degrees of wrist flexion, 17 degrees of radial deviation, and 40 degrees of ulnar deviation. A lack of consensus between these two studies indicates that functional wrist motion varies depending on the activity given and the individual performing the task. Ryu and coworkers[35] went on to conclude that 40 degrees of wrist extension, 40 degrees of wrist flexion, and 40 degrees of combined radioulnar deviation could accomplish most daily activities. The available arc of motion for the radiocarpal prostheses used in wrist arthroplasties range between 40 and 70 degrees of combined wrist flexion-extension and between 20 and 30 degrees of total radioulnar deviation.[7,9,10,21,36–38] This degree of motion is considered sufficient for most patients with arthritis to participate in vocational and avocational activities.

Surgeons may choose from several different wrist prostheses to replace the deteriorated joint. Every prosthesis is unique with regards to surgical approach, allowable arc of motion, and long-term viability. It is important for the treating therapist to be aware of the capabilities of the prosthesis used.

Patients who require wrist arthroplasty often have wrist deformities secondary to soft tissue imbalance.[11] Tenolysis, tendon repair, lengthening, or transfer may be done concurrently with the wrist arthroplasty. Postoperative care, such as splinting, ROM, and length of therapy, may be affected by any one of these interventions. Details of the operative findings, including end-range wrist motion, joint stability, and soft tissue reconstruction, are important in establishing a safe

Fig. 15. Practice sling for positioning thumb CMC extension bridge. Use before making orthosis to assess the correct placement of "bridge." (Copyright Pennsylvania Hand Center, with permission).

Table 2
Thumb CMC arthroplasty with ligament reconstruction with tendon interposition: therapy guidelines

	Immediately Postoperative to 4 Wk Postoperative	4 Wk Postoperative	6 Wk Postoperative	6–8 Wk Postoperative	8–12 Wk Postoperative
Splint	Thumb spica cast (by surgeon)	Forearm-based thumb spica with CMC in extension, MP slight flexion, and IP free. Worn FT except hygiene and controlled AROM.	Splint FT except for light activities, AROM, and hygiene. A neoprene CMC splint may be used for light ADLs instead of the hard splint. Consider a static-progressive CMC extension splint if needed.	Protective splint gradually weaned. Used with increased ADLs and night only.	Splint discontinued.
Therapy	Pain and edema control. AROM of fingers.	Pain and edema control. AROM and AAROM of fingers, and wrist. Thumb AROM in limited range, with metacarpal supported. Begin scar control.	Continue scar control. Increase thumb AROM. Start PROM. Start light thenar strengthening.	Start grip strengthening. Increase resistive exercises but avoid aggressive pinch. Focus on functional strength.	Return to regular activities.
Examples	Ice, elevation, TENS, TGEs, AROM of uninvolved joints.	Thumb metacarpal supported during MP and IP flexion and extension. Active thumb motion for CMC extension, abduction, thumb opposition.	Increased ROM of the thumb. Start thenar strengthening. Modify ADLs.	Progress strengthening as tolerated. Return to hobbies and ADLs as able.	Return to regular activities.
Precautions	Monitor for signs of infection and tight cast.	Avoid active thumb flexion and adduction. Scar thickening.	Avoid painful grip and pinch activities.	Monitor for signs of overuse.	Unrestricted functional use allowed at 12 wk postoperative.

Abbreviations: AAROM, active assisted range of motion; ADLs, activities of daily living; AROM, active range of motion; FT, full time; PROM, passive range of motion; ROM, range of motion; TENS, transcutaneous electrical nerve stimulation; TGE, tendon gliding exercises.

rehabilitation program. By working closely with the surgeon and incorporating the patient's activities and goals, the experienced hand therapist can formulate an optimal treatment plan for each patient after wrist arthroplasty (**Table 3**).

A monitored rehabilitation program emphasizing early motion and low stress to the digits and wrist is necessary to minimize the risk of adhesions and instability.[1,11,39] The following rehabilitation guidelines may require modification depending on the surgeon's preference, the type of prosthesis used, possible soft tissue reconstructions, and the individual's own rate of healing. The hand therapist plays a key role in instructing the patient in the proper progression of care to achieve the desired result of pain-free functional use of the involved wrist.

Three to 10 Days Postoperative

Three to 5 days after surgery, the bulky surgical dressing and cast are removed. A wrist cock-up splint is fabricated to provide the wrist with sufficient support and protection. The forearm-based splint is applied to the anterior aspect of the forearm, with the wrist supported in approximately 0 to 10 degrees of extension and neutral radioulnar deviation (**Fig. 16**). The forearm portion of the splint should be three times the length of the hand portion to adequately protect the surgical site by limiting wrist motion. The patient is educated in edema control, wound care, and splint care. AROM, active-assisted ROM, and placehold exercises are initiated for the digits, wrist, and forearm. The splint is worn full-time except for wrist ROM and hygiene. PROM of the digits is also performed to decrease joint stiffness and prevent adhesions of the extensor tendons and retinaculum.[1,13] Elbow and shoulder AROM exercises are continued. The patient is instructed to do 10 repetitions of each exercise, three to four times per day. If wrist stiffness or adhesions become significant, the frequency is increased for active wrist and digit motion to 10 times every waking hour. Short frequent exercise sessions throughout the day prevent stress to the reconstructed joint while restoring motion.[11] Activity modifications including assistive devices, assistive tools, and alternate ways of accomplishing ADLs should be reviewed with the patient at this time to maximize the patient's independence while providing joint safety.

Ten to 14 Days Postoperative

Sutures are removed around this time. Emphasis is on AROM of all upper extremity joints including the wrist. Pain, edema control and wound care

continue to be a priority. PROM is continued as needed.

Three Weeks Postoperative

AROM exercises are continued, as are pain and edema control. Forearm motion can be introduced at this time. Scar control is started 3 weeks after surgery or 1 week after the incision is completely healed. Scar control is particularly important for incisions at the dorsal wrist because of a high incidence of scar adhesions between skin, extensor tendons, and extensor retinaculum.[1,40] Neuromuscular electric stimulation to the digit and wrist extensors can assist in tendon gliding through the adhered area.[13] Light-resistance putty for digit extension may also improve extensor tendon lags present at MP joint level. Scar control consists of soft tissue mobilization, a pressure pad, and possibly phonophoresis.[13,40] Although no illeffects have been reported, the surgeon should be consulted before doing phonophoresis over the prosthesis because of concerns of breakdown of silicone or plastic components and bone ingrowth with phonophoresis, steroid, or ultrasound use.[12]

Four to 6 Weeks Postoperative

Splint wear can now be decreased to activity only and while sleeping, then discontinued completely by 6 weeks postoperatively. Gentle PROM of the wrist may be started at this time. Excessive force during PROM should be avoided. The use of heat to precondition the tissues helps minimize pain during treatment and maximize the benefits of PROM exercises. Ice after treatment helps to decrease any edema and pain. AROM, edema control, and scar control are continued. The therapist can review joint protection, ADL modifications, and the use of ergonomically designed adaptive aids to encourage long-term viability of the wrist implant. Splint wear is extended if there is any sign of instability. Light gripping resistive exercises may begin now with putty and towel scrunchies (**Fig. 17**).

Six to 8 Weeks Postoperative

More resistive exercises are started approximately 6 to 8 weeks postoperatively. Putty, paper crumble basketball (**Fig. 18**), weight well, Exercise Stik (Anatomy Partners, Atlanta, GA) BTE (Baltimore Therapeutic Equipment Technologies, Inc, Baltimore, MD), grippers, and light weights are some examples of equipment that can be used to improve strength. These exercises can be initiated with very low resistance and gradually increased. Simulating activities that correlate with the

Table 3
Wrist arthroplasty: therapy guidelines

Postoperative	Immediately	5 D	2 Wk	3 Wk	4–6 Wk	6–8 Wk	8–12 Wk
Splint	Bulky postoperative dressing applied.	Wrist cock-up splint FT wear except for hygiene and ROM three times per day.	Continue Splint.	Continue Splint.	Decrease wear to activity only.	Discontinue splint.	Return to regular activities.
Therapy	Pain and edema control. AROM of uninvolved joints.	Pain and edema control. PROM of digits. AROM, TGE and AAROM all joints, including wrist.	Remove sutures.	Begin scar control. Continue AROM and start AAROM of wrist.	Begin gentle PROM of wrist and light resistive exercises. Towel scrunchies.	Continue PROM and AROM. Increase resistive exercises. Focus on functional use of wrist/ADL. Paper crumble-basketball.	
Examples	Ice, elevation, TENS, AROM, TGEs.	TGEs and Place-holds exercises. Ice, elevation, Jobst pump, retrograde massage, compression garments. TENS.	Continue same.	Silicone pads, scar massage, ultrasound, phonophoresis. NMES.	CPM, static-progressive splinting, light PROM. BTE, putty, weight well, functional and light, resistive exercises.	Functional tasks. Increase resistance of strengthening exercises.	
Precautions	Postoperative dressing; skin ulcers Monitor for signs of infection.	Splint fit; signs of infection; nerve compression.	Implant instability.	Scar adhesions	Pain with exercises, resistance, or ROM	No lifting more than 2 lb regularly. lifting more than 10 lb rarely.	Hardware loosening.

Abbreviations: AAROM, active assisted range of motion; ADL, activities of daily living; AROM, active range of motion; BTE, Baltimore Therapeutic equipment; CPM, continuous passive motion machine; FT, full time; HEP, home exercise program; NMES, neuromuscular electric stimulation; PROM, passive range of motion; ROM, range of motion; TENS, transcutaneous electrical nerve stimulation; TGE, tendon gliding exercises.

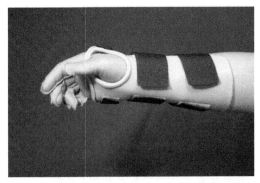

Fig. 16. Wrist forearm-based splint/orthosis (wrist cock-up). An edema glove underneath can improve edema (Copyright Pennsylvania Hand Center, with permission).

patient's lifestyle can help build confidence in the patient's use of the reconstructed wrist. The strengthening program should be reviewed and modified on a weekly basis to improve strength and endurance. AROM, PROM, and scar control are continued.

If joint stiffness persists, a continuous passive motion machine[41] or a static-progressive wrist extension splint may be considered (**Fig. 19**).[1] The force of these devices should be very gentle and tolerable to the patient. The axis of the prosthetic joint needs to be aligned accurately with the continuous passive motion machine or splint to avoid stress on the implant. The continuous passive motion machine and static-progressive splint may be started three times per day for 30-minute sessions and increased or decreased depending on the patient's tolerance and progress. For best results, follow PROM with AROM because at that point the joint is primed and capable of achieving greater active range.

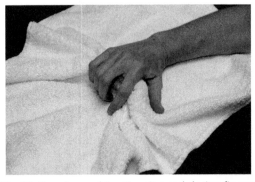

Fig. 17. Towel scrunchies. Opening and closing fingers around a towel encourages tendon gliding with a little resistance (Copyright Pennsylvania Hand Center, with permission).

Eight to 12 Weeks Postoperative

Most patients complete therapy approximately 3 months after surgery.[11] A final assessment using the DASH, QuickDASH,[16] or Patient Rated Wrist Evaluation[17] on the patient's last visit allows for an objective comparison of function before and after surgery. Final scores on these questionnaires should place the patient within the "mild-difficulties" range regarding ADLs. Painless adequate function, motion, and moderate grip strength is the ultimate goal. All measurements should be improved when compared with preoperative measurements.[9,21,38,42,43]

THERAPY AFTER DRUJ ARTHROPLASTY

DRUJ arthroplasty is a salvage procedure performed in cases of trauma, deformity, osteoarthritis, inflammatory disease, or a failed previous DRUJ surgery.[44] It is a last resort to preserve joint function, relieve pain, and avoid fusion. These patients undergo surgery if forearm rotation and grip activities have become extremely painful and limited. Arthritis between the radius and ulna at the sigmoid notch or impingement because of a positive ulnar variance is usually the cause of pain. DRUJ arthroplasties are intended for patients with low functional demands because joint stability is often compromised in the effort to restore pain-free forearm rotation.[44] Procedures to improve joint stability and maximize strength after DRUJ arthroplasty are presently being investigated.[42,45,46]

Various Procedures

DRUJ arthroplasties are named and categorized according to procedure type. Resection of the ulnar head is called the Darrach procedure. Although pain is reduced with this procedure, the stabilizing ligaments are resected causing poor load-bearing and grip strength. Therefore, variations on this procedure and partial resections were developed. The Bowers hemiresection-interposition technique is a resection of the ulnar head where it articulates with the radius.[47] The Watson matched resection is similar with the goal being to remove the arthritic joint while preserving the ligaments that stabilize forearm rotation.[47,48] The Feldon wafer procedure resects the distal ulna while leaving the radioulnar joint and its ligaments intact.[47] It is used in cases of positive ulnar variance with minimum arthritis at the sigmoid notch. Ulna shortening, as described by Milch, allows for the most stable load-bearing articulation because the surgery does not disrupt the ligaments involved in forearm rotation.[47] Fusion of the distal radius and ulna to create a more proximal pseudojoint at the ulnar shaft was described by

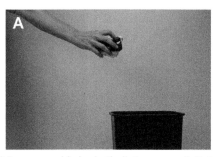
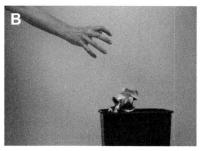

Fig. 18. (*A, B*) Paper crumble basketball. Improves digit dexterity and gliding with light resistance and functional wrist motion (Copyright Pennsylvania Hand Center, with permission).

Sauvé and Kapandji. All these procedures are attempts to provide a stable joint with pain-free functional rotation and grip.

Most studies acknowledge that the ulnar head is important in preserving strength and stability during forearm rotation.[45] They agree that the biomechanics of the forearm make it prone to instability if the anatomy is altered.[45,48] As a result, ulnar head replacements, such as the Swanson silicone, Herbert, and U-head, became popular.[44,45,49] In 1988, the first DRUJ hemiarthroplasty was introduced and later in 2004, the total DRUJ joint replacement was developed.[50,51] More recently, a DRUJ prosthesis including an ulna and radial sigmoid notch component became available.[46] Hardware continues to evolve to better simulate the original anatomy and achieve stability, osseointegration, motion, and strength.[45,46,52]

The choice of a procedure depends on several factors. These include the severity of the cartilage and soft tissue damage at the DRUJ, and the desired results and activity level of the patient. Pain with forearm rotation is most likely caused by impingement at the sigmoid notch with a patient history of trauma, inflammatory arthritis, or a congenital deformity.[49] The most common DRUJ arthroplasty is the matched resection arthroplasty. Some surgeons do not like the matched resection arthroplasty, arguing that axial stability is lost with removal of the ulna head.[47,53] The stability of the DRUJ may be compromised because of convergence of the radius and ulna, especially with grip and forearm rotation.

Pain-free stable forearm rotation and grip while maintaining normal wrist motion is the main goal of therapy after DRUJ arthroplasty (**Table 4**). After surgery, the wrist and forearm may be immobilized for a full 6 weeks. This is followed by progressive motion of the reconstructed DRUJ. After functional pain-free ROM is achieved, strengthening is introduced. The immediate rehabilitation goals are to decrease edema and pain. Long-term goals include increased pain-free forearm rotation, wrist motion, grip strength, weight bearing, and ADL performance.[49]

Immediately Postoperative

The patient is casted postoperatively for 2 to 6 weeks to promote stability. A short- or long-arm cast preventing wrist and forearm motion may be applied by the surgeon. The cast is used longer in patients whose priority is stability. While the forearm and wrist are immobilized, motion of digits, elbow, and shoulder is important to reduce edema and pain and improve circulation. After cast removal, if forearm rotation is not detrimental to surgery, a forearm-based bivalve wrist splint is fabricated with the wrist in 10 to 20 degrees of extension to minimize wrist motion and allow use of the involved hand (**Fig. 20**). For patients requiring restrictions in forearm rotation, a sugar-tong (**Fig. 21**) or Muenster splint is fabricated (**Fig. 22**). ADL modifications are made to maximize independence. Scar control is initiated 1 to 2 weeks after suture removal.

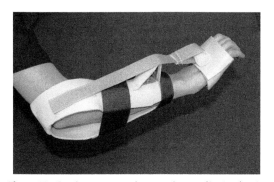

Fig. 19. Static progressive wrist splint/orthosis. Forearm-base around elbow prevents distal migration and hand piece with Velcro attachment allows for controlled wrist extension (shown) and wrist flexion (not shown) (Copyright Pennsylvania Hand Center, with permission).

Table 4
DRUJ arthroplasty: therapy guidelines

Postoperative	Immediately	10–14 D	2–6 Wk	6–8 Wk	6–12 Wk
Splint	Bulky postoperative dressing/cast applied.	Wrist bi-valve splint or Sugartong or Muenster splint FT wear	Splint FT except AROM and hygiene. Start AROM of wrist and forearm	Decrease splint use. Wear with increased ADL, and night. Add static progressive sup/pron sling if needed	Discontinue protective splint. Continue sup/pron sling until rotation full
Therapy	Pain and edema control. AROM of uninvolved joints. ADL assessment and modifications	Pain and edema control. AROM of uninvolved joints. Sutures out.	Start AROM and AAROM wrist and forearm. Start scar control	Start PROM and gradual strengthening of wrist and forearm	Return to regular activities. Modify ADLs as needed.
Examples	Ice, elevation, TENS, AROM uninvolved joints	TGEs, TENS, ice, elevation, Jobst pump, retrograde massage, compression garments.	Towel scrunches, Nonresistive exercises, such as BTE and weight well. Silicone pads, scar massage, ultrasound, phonophoresis.	CPM, static-progressive splinting, PROM. BTE, gripper, weight well, hammer stretch, functional and light resistive exercises.	Increase resistance of strengthening exercises. Incorporate patient's activity inventory and hobbies. Return to patient lifestyle.
Precautions	Postoperative dressing; skin ulcers. Monitor for signs of infection. No forearm or wrist ROM	Splint fit; signs of infection; nerve compression.	Implant instability. Scar adhesions	Pain with exercises, resistance or ROM	ADLs reviewed/modified. Hardware loosening.

Abbreviations: AAROM, active assisted range of motion; ADL, activities of daily living; AROM, active range of motion; BTE, Baltimore Therapeutic Equipment; CPM, continuous passive motion machine; FT, full time; PROM, passive range of motion; ROM, range of motion; Sup/Pron, supination/pronation; TENS, transcutaneous electrical nerve stimulation; TGE, tendon gliding exercises.

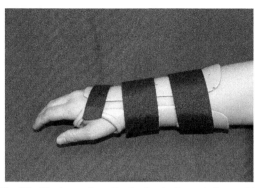

Fig. 20. Bivalve wrist splint/orthosis. Dorsal piece with a wrist forearm-based orthosis provides additional support (Copyright Pennsylvania Hand Center, with permission).

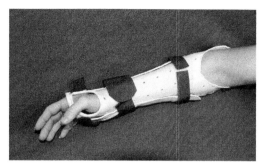

Fig. 22. Muenster splint. Prevents forearm rotation and allows for some elbow flexion (Copyright Pennsylvania Hand Center, with permission).

Two to 6 Weeks Postoperative

When the joint is deemed stable by the surgeon, usually between 2 and 6 weeks postoperatively, the splint is removed for hygiene and light AROM of the wrist and forearm. A BTE program may be used without resistance for AROM of the wrist and forearm within pain-free limitations. Scar control and edema control techniques are continued.

Six to 12 Weeks Postoperative

At this time, the splint is weaned during sedentary activities and continued with heavier activities and while sleeping. Progressive strengthening and passive forearm rotation are started. A BTE program, weight well, putty, and gripper with gradually increased resistance can improve functional strength within a pain-free range. Holding a hammer in rotation with the elbow close to the body provides a stretch to improve forearm motion and load tolerance (**Fig. 23**A). Moving the patient's hand closer to

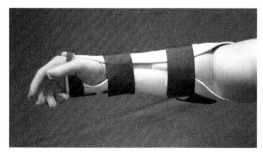

Fig. 21. Sugar-tong splint. Prevents forearm rotation by including the elbow. When fabricating, avoid bony prominences, such as the medial and lateral epicondyles (Copyright Pennsylvania Hand Center, with permission).

the end of the hammer's handle increases leverage and gives the patient encouragement as pain-free function increases (**Fig. 23**B).[15]

The forearm derotation sling is a static-progressive splint that can be fabricated to gently increase forearm pronation and supination.[15] In a modified fabrication from our original description in 1996, it can be made from the patient's protective wrist splint and a long piece of 2-in wide Velcro loop (**Fig. 24**). The Velcro is worn around the patient's neck with one end attached to hook-Velcro on the proximal end of the splint and the other end attached to hook-Velcro on the distal end of the splint. This "sling" should allow the patient's elbow to relax at a 90 degrees when sitting in an armless chair or standing. Before each end of the long loop-Velcro is attached to the splint, it is wrapped around the splint to create a rotational force in supination (**Fig. 24**A) or pronation (**Fig. 24**B). Initially, gravity and the weight of the patient's arm provide the torque needed to rotate the forearm and improve motion. Later on, weight may be added: a 12-in long Velcro is attached to the most distal end of the splint to carry a 1- to 3-lb weight (**Fig. 24**C). This extra weight hangs from the splint to encourage either pronation or supination if gravity alone is not sufficient. The patient is instructed to wear the splint 20 to 30 minutes at a time, three to four times a day as tolerated. The splint and strengthening and PROM should be pain-free. At 12 to 16 weeks postoperatively, the splint is discontinued and the patient can return to normal activities.

Therapy Results

Functional and subjective outcomes after DRUJ arthroplasty vary. Complications may include residual pain secondary to impingement, recurrent instability, or weakness.[45] Other complications include hardware loosening, infection, nerve injury,

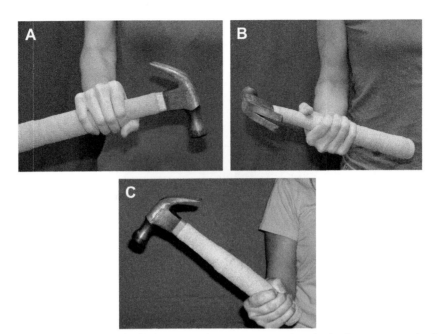

Fig. 23. Hammer stretch can be used to encourage forearm rotation (*A, B*). The hammer can also be used for strengthening, by moving the hand closer to the handle end (*C*) (Copyright Pennsylvania Hand Center, with permission).

tendonitis, and limited motion.[53] Partial or total resection of the distal ulna usually resolves the primary complaint of pain but with limited motion and strength in the involved wrist and forearm. With recent improvements in DRUJ hardware, patients report improved grip strength, weight bearing capabilities, good pain relief, and satisfaction with the procedure.[45,49] These results are from short-term follow-up studies of less than 2 years. The long-term effectiveness and life span of DRUJ replacement arthroplasties are not yet known.

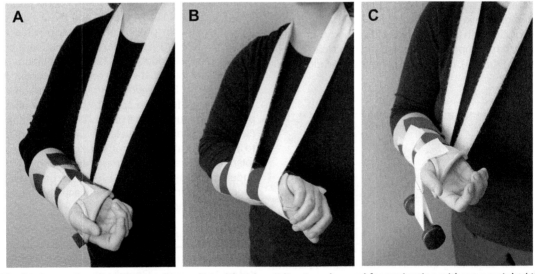

Fig. 24. Derotation sling. Wrist cock-up splint with Velcro "sling" can be used for supination without a weight (*A*) or for pronation (*B*). Notice the sling's placement onto the radial side of the splint determines the direction of the rotational force. A weight may be added for more torque (*C*) (Copyright Pennsylvania Hand Center, with permission).

SUMMARY

Although arthroplasties continue to evolve with advancing technology, rehabilitation goals remain the same: a painless, stable joint capable of functional motion and adequate strength during everyday activities. With new developments, eventually the durability of these reconstructions may improve. This would allow patients to undergo arthroplasty surgery with the hope of once again fully participating in all their previous hobbies, including sports and more demanding activities. Restoring the reconstructed extremity completely to full capacity would be a great achievement and is the ultimate desire of all hand surgeons and therapists who work with this patient population.

ACKNOWLEDGMENTS

The authors acknowledge the contributions of Marwan A. Wehbe, MD, to splint design and the treatment protocols described in this article.

REFERENCES

1. Adams BD. Complications of wrist arthroplasty. Hand Clin 2010;26:213–20.
2. Huang KM, Naidu SH. Total wrist arthroplasty: is there a role? Curr Opin Orthop 2002;13:260–8.
3. Lawler EA, Paksima N. Total wrist arthroplasty. Bull NYU Hosp Jt Dis 2006;64(3–4):98–105.
4. Anderson MC, Adams BD. Total wrist arthroplasty. Hand Clin 2005;21:621–30.
5. Carlson JR, Simmons BP. Total wrist arthroplasty. J Am Acad Orthop Surg 1998;6(5):308–15.
6. Lorei MP, Figgie MP, Ranawat CS, et al. Failed total wrist arthroplasty. Analysis of failures and results of operative management. Clin Orthop Relat Res 1997;(342):84–93.
7. Meuli HC. Total wrist arthroplasty. Clin Orthop Relat Res 1997;342:77–83.
8. Trieb K. Treatments of the wrist in rheumatoid arthritis. J Hand Surg Am 2008;33(A):113–23.
9. Kozin SH. Arthroplasty of the hand and wrist: a surgeon's perspective. J Hand Ther 1999;12(2):123–32.
10. Kirkpatrick WH, Kozin SH, Uhl RL. Early motion after arthroplasty. Hand Clin 1996;12(1):73–86.
11. Lockard MA. Implications for rehabilitation after total wrist arthroplasty. Tech Hand Up Extrem Surg 2004;8(3):138–41.
12. Michlovitz S. Arthroplasty of the hand and wrist: therapist's commentary. J Hand Ther 1999;13(2):133–4.
13. Burke SL. Scar management. In: Hand and upper extremity rehabilitation: a practical guide. 3rd edition. St Louis (MO): Elsevier Churchill Livingstone; 2006. p. 39–50.
14. Wehbe MA. Tendon gliding exercises. Am J Occup Ther 1987;41:164–7.
15. Wehbe MA. Early motion after hand wrist reconstruction. Hand Clin 1996;12(1):25–9.
16. Solway S, Beaton DE, McConnell S, et al. The dash outcome measure user's manual. 2nd edition. Toronto: Institute for Work & Health; 2002.
17. MacDermid JC. Development of a scale for patient rating of wrist pain and disability. J Hand Ther 1996;9:178–83.
18. Wong JY. The use of disabilities of the arm shoulder and hand questionnaire in rehabilitation after acute traumatic hand injuries. J Hand Ther 2007;20(1):49–55.
19. Clinical assessment recommendations. 2nd edition. Chicago: American Society of Hand Therapists; 1992.
20. Cambridge-Keeling CA. Range-of-motion measurement of the hand. In: Mackin EJ, Callahan AD, Skirven TM, et al, editors. Rehabilitation of the hand and upper extremity, vol. 1, 5th edition. Philadelphia: Mosby, Inc; 2002. p. 169–82.
21. Rizzo M, Beckenbaugh RD. Results of biaxial total wrist arthroplasty with a modified (long) metacarpal stem. J Hand Surg Am 2003;28(4):577–84.
22. Sardelli M, Tashjian RZ, MacWilliams BA. Functional elbow range of motion for contemporary tasks. J Bone Joint Surg Am 2011;93(5):471–7.
23. Cooney W, Chao E. Biomechanical analysis of static forces in the thumb during hand function. J Bone Joint Surg Am 1977;59(1):27–36.
24. Gehrmann S, Tang J, Li Z, et al. Motion deficit of the thumb in CMC joint arthritis. J Hand Surg Am 2010;35(9):1449–53.
25. Poole J, Pellegrini V. Arthritis of the thumb basal joint complex. J Hand Ther 2000;13(1):91–107.
26. Menon J. The problem of trapeziometacarpal degenerative arthritis. Clin Orthop Relat Res 1983;175:155–65.
27. Landsmeer J. The coordination of finger joint motions. J Bone Joint Surg Am 1963;459(8):1654–62.
28. Wilder F, Barrett J, Farina E. Joint-specific prevalence of osteoarthritis of the hand. Osteoarthritis Cartilage 2006;14(9):953–7.
29. Van Heest A, Kallemeier P. Thumb carpal metacarpal arthritis. J Am Acad Orthop Surg 2008;16(3):140–51.
30. Amadio P, Millender L, Smith R. Silicone spacer or tendon spacer for trapezium resection arthroplasty: comparison of results. J Hand Surg 1982;7:237–44.
31. Burton R, Pellegrini V. Surgical management of basal joint arthritis of the thumb. Part II. Ligament reconstruction with tendon interposition arthroplasty. J Hand Surg 1986;11(A):324–32.
32. Yang S, Weiland A. First metacarpal subsidence during pinch after ligament reconstruction and tendon interposition basal joint arthroplasty of the thumb. J Hand Surg Am 1998;23(5):879–83.
33. Saunders R. Thumb carpometacarpal joint arthroplasty. In: Burke S, Higgins J, McClinton M, et al,

editors. Hand and upper extremity rehabilitation: a practical guide. Philadelphia: Elsevier, Inc; 2006. p. 617–23.

34. Palmer AK, Werner FW, Murphy D, et al. Functional wrist motion: a biomechanics study. J Hand Surg Am 1985;10(1):39–46.

35. Ryu J, Cooney WP, Askew LJ, et al. Functional ranges of motion of the wrist joint. J Hand Surg Am 1991;16(3):409–19.

36. Strunk S, Gracker W. Wrist joint arthroplasty: results after 41 prostheses. Handchir Mikrochir Plast Chir 2009;4(3):141–7.

37. Adams BD. Total wrist arthroplasty. Tech Hand Up Extrem Surg 2004;8(3):130–7.

38. Radmer S, Andersen R, Sparmann M. Wrist arthroplasty with a new generation of prostheses in patients with rheumatoid arthritis. J Hand Surg Am 1999;24(5):935–43.

39. Divelbiss BJ, Sollerman C, Adams BD. Early results of the total wrist arthroplasty in rheumatoid arthritis. J Hand Surg 2002;27(2):195–204.

40. Crosby CA, Wehbe MA. Early motion protocols in hand and wrist rehabilitation. Hand Clin 1996;12:31–41.

41. Salter RB. History of rest and motion and the scientific basis for early continuous passive motion. Hand Clin 1996;12:1–11.

42. Cobb TK, Beckenbaugh RD. Biaxial total-wrist arthroplasty. J Hand Surg Am 1996;21(6):1011–21.

43. Stegeman M, Rijnberg WJ, van Loon CJ. Biaxial total wrist arthroplasty in rheumatoid arthritis. Satisfactory functional results. Rheumatol Int 2005;25:191–4.

44. Herbert T, van Schoonhoven J. Ulnar head replacement. Tech Hand Up Extrem Surg 2007;11(1):98–108.

45. Laurentin-Perez L, Goodwin A, Babb B, et al. A study of functional outcomes following implantation of a total distal radioulnar joint prosthesis. J Hand Surg Eur Vol 2008;33:18–28.

46. Surgical technique stability PGT sigmoid notch total DRUJ system. Morrisville (PA): Small Bone Innovations; 2006.

47. Bowers W. Distal radioulnar joint arthroplasty: current concepts. Clin Orthop Relat Res 1992;275:104–9.

48. Tsai P, Paksima N. The distal radioulnar joint. Bull NYU Hosp Jt Dis 2009;67(1):90–6.

49. Kaiser K, Bodell L, Berger R. Functional outcomes after arthroplasty of the distal radioulnar joint and hand therapy: a case series. J Hand Ther 2008;21:398–407.

50. Wehbé MA. Pitfalls of radio-ulnar joint injuries. Presented at the Jefferson Orthopaedic Society Annual Meeting. Philadelphia, November 15, 1991.

51. Wehbé MA. Pitfalls of radio-ulnar joint injuries. Presented at the Symposium American Society for Surgery of the Hand Annual Meeting. Phoenix, November 13, 1992.

52. Surgical technique uhead ulnar implant system. Morrisville (PA): Small Bone Innovations; 2008.

53. Sauder D, King G. Hemiarthroplasty of the distal ulna with an eccentric prosthesis. Tech Hand Up Extrem Surg 2007;11(1):115–20.

A Carpal Ligament Substitute
Part 1: Polyester Suture

John A. Martin Jr, MD[a,b], Marwan A. Wehbé, MD[c,d],*

KEYWORDS

- Carpal ligament • Scapholunate • Triquetrolunate • Lunotriquetral • Mersilene • Wrist ligament
- Ligament substitute

KEY POINTS

- Four loops of 2-0 polyester fiber suture (Mersilene) were found to exceed the ultimate tensile strength of the scapholunate interosseous ligament.
- This construct approximates a normal ligament stress/strain curve and can theoretically facilitate fibrous tissue ingrowth.
- The authors recommend the use of polyester suture in the reconstruction of carpal and other ligaments.

INTRODUCTION

Primary repair and reconstruction of the scapholunate ligament are difficult and the reported results inconsistent.[1–3] Reconstruction may be complicated by absence of reparable tissues, particularly in chronic ligament insufficiency. Therefore, augmentation or substitution of the scapholunate ligament complex is a conceptually attractive alternative. The size and relationship of the carpal bones, however, impose many technical constraints on ligament substitution. An ideal ligament substitute would approximate the native ligament biomechanically, be readily available and inexpensive, provide potential for fibrous tissue ingrowth, and be easy to use.

The authors propose the use of polyester fiber sutures as a substitute for the scapholunate and other ligaments. This article addresses the in vitro mechanical properties of this potential ligament substitute.

METHODS

All sutures were tested in tension to failure on a stress-testing machine (Instron Model 1000, Instron, Canton, Massachusetts). S-hooks were used for couplers to which the sutures were attached. The following sutures were tested: Ethibond 2-0, 3-0, and 4-0 (Ethicon, Somerville, New Jersey), Mersilene 2-0 and 3-0 (Ethicon), and Cottony Dacron No. 1 (Deknatel, Fall River, Massachusetts). These sutures are all made with nonabsorbable braided multifilaments of polyester fiber (polyethylene-terephthalate). Such sutures have been shown to elicit some degree of inflammatory reaction and fibrous tissue ingrowth in vivo.[4] Their tensile strength in vivo is apparently indefinite.[5]

Ethibond and Mersilene are essentially the same suture material with the exception of the polybutilate coating used on Ethibond. Polybutilate is a polymer lubricant material that adheres strongly to the polyester fiber. It is nonabsorbable and inert and does not affect the tensile strength of the suture. It acts to reduce the coefficient of friction during passage of suture through tissue. It also seals the space between the suture fibers and prevents tissue ingrowth.

Cottony Dacron has also the same material and construction as Mersilene. It undergoes an additional step in manufacture, however, called

[a] Commonwealth Sports Medicine, Reading, PA, USA; [b] St. Joseph Medical Center, Reading, PA, USA;
[c] Pennsylvania Hand Center, 101 South Bryn Mawr Avenue, Suite 300, Bryn Mawr, PA 19010, USA;
[d] Jefferson Medical College, Philadelphia, PA, USA
* Corresponding author. Pennsylvania Hand Center, 101 South Bryn Mawr Avenue, Suite 300, Bryn Mawr, PA 19010.
E-mail address: Marwan.Wehbe@pahandcenter.com

Hand Clin 29 (2013) 143–148
http://dx.doi.org/10.1016/j.hcl.2012.08.026
0749-0712/13/$ – see front matter © 2013 Elsevier Inc. All rights reserved.

mechanical softening. This procedure yields a softer, less stiff character to the suture. With less stiffness, there is less tendency for a braided structure to open spontaneously.[4] Such a property would interfere with fibrous ingrowth. A stiffer braided structure is preferred when ingrowth is desirable. Mersilene is, therefore, a logical choice because it is uncoated and not mechanically softened.

Each trial was performed in the following manner. The S-hooks were positioned 2 cm apart. One loop of suture (2 strands of material) was placed around the S-hooks and tied to itself with a surgeon's knot followed by 2 standard throws in a square fashion, to prevent knot slippage. Knot integrity was confirmed for each trial by inspection. In addition, the stress/strain curves were reviewed after each trial to identify any abrupt increase in length of the suture loops before strand failure denoting knot slippage. A submaximal peak in the curve indicated suture length change, indicating knot slippage (**Fig. 1**). Each trial

was continued to failure. Data were obtained for 1 to 4 loops of each suture evaluated. Loops were created by passing one strand of suture continuously around the S-hooks the appropriate number of times, ending with a single knot per trial.

To account for slack in the suture loops and the weight of the hooks, a starting stress of 10 N was designated as point zero. Each suture was tested at a strain rate of 5 mm/min and 100 mm/min to determine if appreciable viscoelastic properties were present. This range of strain rates has been reported in a study of the viscoelastic properties of human scapholunate ligaments.[6]

Trials were performed using increasing number of suture loops until the physiologic range, previously identified by Mayfield and Williams[7] as 350 N to 400 N, was exceeded. Further data were obtained on several other suture sizes at 2 different strain rates to determine if significant viscoelastic behavior was present in potential ligament substitutes. For this, several trials of 1 to 4 loops of various sutures were performed at 5 mm/min and

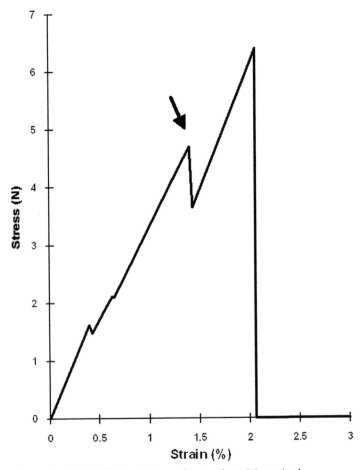

Fig. 1. Knot slippage (*arrow*) with 2-0 Ethibond suture (3 strands at 5.0 mm/sec).

100 mm/min. Those sutures with an ultimate tensile strength within the physiologic range were then tested again for 10 trials at 50 mm/min strain rate, because this was the approximate rate used by Mayfield and Williams.[7]

RESULTS

When examining the data of different loading rates, there seems no significant difference in the ultimate tensile strength between the 2 strain rates tested (**Table 1**).

Three sutures were found to have a tensile strength exceeding that of the human scapholunate ligament of 359 N. Four loops of Ethibond 2-0, 4 loops of Mersilene 2-0, and 3 loops of 3-mm Cottony Dacron suture (see **Table 1**). Further trials with Cottony Dacron were not done because the large size and bulkiness of its 3 loops limit its usefulness as a scapholunate ligament substitute. Ten further trials of both Ethibond 2-0 and Mersilene 2-0 were performed (**Table 2**).

The mean tensile strength for 4 loops of Ethibond 2-0 was 410 N (range 393–435 N). The mean strain was 3.8 mm (range 3.3–4.3 mm) at 50-mm/min strain rate. Mean tensile strength of 4 loops of Mersilene 2-0 was 404 N (range 373–440 N), with a mean strain of 3.6 mm (range 3.2–4.0 mm) at 50 mm/min loading rate.

DISCUSSION

Failure of carpal ligaments can have disastrous effects.[1,8] Late reconstruction, by direct suture and with tendon grafts or tendon transfers, has not proved successful with any consistency.[1,2] For these reasons, investigation of the biomechanics of normal intercarpal ligaments and possible substitutes became essential.

Logan and colleagues[6] reported a 70% increase in stiffness in the scapholunate ligament, with an increase in strain rate from 5.0 mm/min to 100 mm/min. Our tested sutures did not, however, behave in a similar fashion; there was no significant difference between the 2 loading rates. This makes the suture substitute equally reliable at any of these loading rates.

Mayfield and Williams[7] found the scapholunate interosseous ligament to be the strongest of the intercarpal ligaments. They also demonstrated midsubstance failure of the scapholunate ligament in the majority of specimens at 359 N.[7] The suture material and configuration that we have identified, therefore, exceed the ultimate tensile strength of fresh human interosseous carpal ligaments.

Many prosthetic ligaments have been evaluated in the past and include carbon fiber,[9–11] polytetrafluoroethylene (Gore-Tex[12]), braided polyester tape (Dacron[13]), polypropylene,[14] polyester fiber or glass,[15] and xenografts.[16] Most of the materials

Table 1
Suture stress/strain values at varying strain rates

Suture	Loops	Stress (N)		Strain (mm)	
		5 mm/min	l00 mm/min	5 mm/min	l00 mm/min
Ethibond 2-0	1	73	—	4.5	—
	2	160	—	4.4	—
	3	269	—	6.7	—
	4	356	—	7.3	—
Ethibond 4-0	1	24.5	23.5	4.3	3.2
	2	60	57.9	2.5	5.2
	3	108.9	89.2	3.0	3.0
	4	142	129.8	4.2	2.8
Mersilene 2-0	1	53	—	2.0	—
	2	149	—	2.8	—
	3	246	—	2.8	—
	4	377	367	3.4	3.5
Mersilene 3-0	1	37.8	39.9	3.2	2.7
	2	85.5	119.6	2.8	3.0
	3	145.1	148.9	1.9	2.6
	4	195	148.9	2.0	—
Cottony Dacron No.1	1	108	106	8.3	6.9
	2	227	286	5.0	4.5
	3	380	462	5.8	5.0

Table 2
Stress/strain data of proposed scapholunate ligament substitute (strain rate 50 mm/min)

Suture[a]	Stress (N)		Strain (mm)	
	Mean	Range	Mean	Range
Mersilene	404	373–440	3.6	3.2–4.0
Ethibond	410	393–435	3.8	3.3–4.3

[a] 4 Loops 2-0 caliber; 10 trials for each suture.

are biologically inert and allow for fibrous tissue and collagen ingrowth.[11–14] Gore-Tex, Dacron, and carbon fiber have been successfully used in humans for substitution or augmentation of the anterior cruciate, coracoacromial, and ankle ligaments.[12,17,18]

The physical and biologic characteristics of these materials are appealing for scapholunate ligament reconstruction. Most may be excluded on the basis of their large size or certain physical properties. For example, the Gore-Tex ligament is approximately 1 cm in diameter; it is composed of a single continuous fiber; therefore, cutting or trimming the prosthesis to the appropriate size is not possible. The Dacron ligament is also unsuitable, because of a large diameter (8 mm); it cannot be trimmed because of its design of internal Dacron tapes and woven velour cover.

Carbon fiber has been shown to allow tissue ingrowth in repaired ligaments.[19–21] It is brittle, however, tends to fragment, and can produce a localized synovitis.[13,22,23] Furthermore, carbon fragments have been isolated from regional lymph nodes adjacent to the area of reconstruction.[10]

Tissue ingrowth has been shown, in implantation studies, to occur within polyester fibers and Gore-Tex.[12,13,15] This allows for improved bonding of the suture to surrounding tissue with the lapse of time. Furthermore, the polyester-fibrous tissue complex has been shown to more closely approximate the stress-strain pattern of normal tendon (**Fig. 2**).

The polyester filament-tissue complex has been shown to be stiffer than intact tendon in the rabbit.[15] This increase in stiffness is attributed to the polyester fiber and not the ingrown fibrous tissue; synthetic materials are much stiffer than intact tendon and, therefore, show negligible change in length at low loads (**Fig. 3**). This inherent stiffness of the polyester-fibrous tissue complex is useful in reconstructive surgery. Specifically, the length of the reconstructive ligament can be determined at surgery, anticipating little postoperative

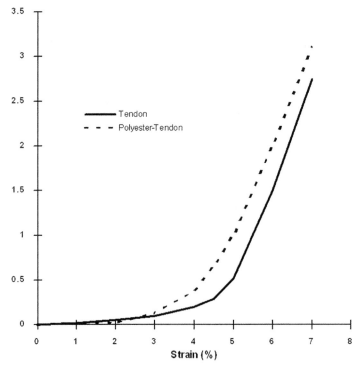

Fig. 2. Stress/strain curves of rabbit Achilles tendon and polyester fiber with collagen ingrowth composite. (*Adapted from* Goodship AE, Wilcock SA, Shah JS. The development of tissue around various prosthetic implants used as replacements for ligaments and tendons. Clin Orthop Relat Res 1985;196:61–8.)

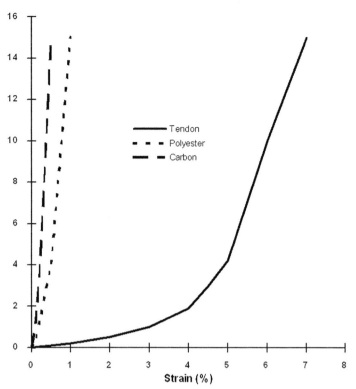

Fig. 3. Stress/strain curves of carbon, polyester, and tendon collagen fibers. (*Adapted from* Goodship AE, Wilcock SA, Shah JS. The development of tissue around various prosthetic implants used as replacements for ligaments and tendons. Clin Orthop Relat Res 1985;196:61–8.)

change. Fibrous ingrowth provides strength to the construct and assumes greater load absorption with time, because the suture possibly weakens from fatigue failure.

The multistrand, braided construction of polyester fiber sutures has 3 other important characteristics. First, the braided construction of multiple single strands, configured in several loops at surgery, provides a much greater surface area available for ingrowth compared with monofilament suture. Second, the braided construct is easier to handle than monofilament types. As a result, braided sutures are less susceptible to damage by kinking and crushing, which would otherwise weaken the suture and may lead to breakage.[4,24] Finally, knot security is higher for Mersilene than many other polyester sutures.[25]

In vivo, axial loading of the palm with the wrist extended (as in a fall on the outstretched hand) applies tension to the interosseous scapholunate ligament complex.[26] When its ultimate tensile strength is exceeded, failure of the ligament or ligament-bone junction occurs. Therefore, the ultimate tensile strength is one of the most important characteristics of a scapholunate ligament substitute. In addition, the ligament substitute must bear physiologic loads until tissue ingrowth and

collagen reorganization occur. Such ingrowth is facilitated by the large surface area of multifilament braided structure of 4 loops of material.

The mode of failure between Ethibond and Mersilene seemed slightly different. The 2-0 Ethibond consistently failed in midstrand. In contrast the Mersilene suture consistently failed at the suture knot junction, implying cutting of the strand by the knot. Because both sutures are made of braided polyester fiber, it is possible that the polybutilate coating of the Ethibond suture is responsible for the difference. Given the mean ultimate tensile strength of the 2 sutures differed by only 6 N and strain rates differed by 0.2 mm, it is unlikely that this finding represents a clinically significant difference.

In summary, we have found that Mersilene is a candidate for reconstruction of carpal ligaments on theoretic grounds. Four continuous loops of Mersilene exceed the ultimate tensile strength of human interosseous scapholunate ligament. No appreciable viscoelastic properties were identified. Therefore, the authors conclude that 4 loops of 2-0 Mersilene suture could substitute for a functionally absent scapholunate ligament. A clinical trial of such a reconstruction, with encouraging results, is described in Part 2 of this chapter.

REFERENCES

1. Dobyns JH, Linscheid RL, Chao EY, et al. Traumatic instability of the wrist. American Academy of Orthopaedic Surgeons. Inst Course Lect 1975;24:182–99.
2. Glickel SZ, Millender LH. Ligamentous reconstruction for chronic intercarpal instability. J Hand Surg 1984;9A:514–27.
3. Green DP. Carpal dislocations and instabilities. In: Green DP, editor. Operative hand surgery, vol. 2, 2nd edition. New York: Churchill Livingston; 1988. p. 917.
4. Roy J. Cardiovascular sutures electron microscopy. Scanning Electron Microsc 1980;3:204.
5. Wound closure manual. New Jersey: Ethicon Inc; 1985. p. 22, 24, 25, 90.
6. Logan SE, Nowak MD, Gould PL, et al. Biomechanical behavior of the scapholunate ligament. Biomed Sci Instrum 1986;22:81–5.
7. Mayfield JK, Williams WJ. Biomechanical properties of human carpal ligaments. Orthop Trans 1979;3:143–4.
8. Blevens AD, Light TR, Jablonsky WS, et al. Radiocarpal articular contact characteristics with scaphoid instability. J Hand Surg Am 1989;14:781–90.
9. Claes L, Neugelbauer R. In vivo and in vitro investigation of the long-term behavior and fatigue strength of carbon fiber ligament replacement. Clin Orthop Relat Res 1985;196:99–111.
10. Forster IW, Ralis ZA, McKibbin B, et al. Biological reaction to carbon fiber implants. Clin Orthop Relat Res 1978;131:299–307.
11. Mendes DG, Iusim M, Angel D, et al. Histologic pattern of biomechanical properties of the carbon fiber-augmented ligament tendon. Clin Orthop Relat Res 1985;196:51–60.
12. Bolton CW, Bruchman WC. The Gore-Tex expanded polytetrafluoroethylene prosthetic ligament. Clin Orthop Relat Res 1985;196:202–13.
13. Park JP, Grana WA, Chitwood JS. A high strength Dacron augmentation for cruciate ligament reconstruction. Clin Orthop Relat Res 1985;196:175–85.
14. McPherson GK, Mendenhall HV, Gibbons DF, et al. Experimental mechanical and histologic evaluation of the Kennedy ligament augmentation device. Clin Orthop Relat Res 1985;196:186–95.
15. Goodship AE, Wilcock SA, Shah JS. The development of tissue around various prosthetic implants used as replacements for ligaments and tendons. Clin Orthop Relat Res 1985;196:61–8.
16. McMaster WC. A histologic assessment of canine anterior cruciate substitution with bovine xenograft. Clin Orthop Relat Res 1985;196:196–201.
17. Kappakas GS, McMaster JH. Repair of acromioclavicular separation using a Dacron prosthesis graft. Clin Orthop Relat Res 1978;131:247–51.
18. Park JP, Arnold JA, Coker TP, et al. Lateral ligamentous reconstruction of the unstable ankle with Dacron. A preliminary report. Presented at the Annual Meeting of the Am Orthop Soc for Sports Med. Lake Tahoe, June 21–25, 1981.
19. Jenkins DH. The repair of cruciate ligament with flexible carbon fibre: a longer term study of the indication of new ligaments and of the fate of the implanted carbon. J Bone Joint Surg Br 1978;60:520–2.
20. Jenkins DH. Ligament induction by filamentous carbon fiber. Clin Orthop Relat Res 1985;196:86–7.
21. Lemaire M. Reinforcement of tendons and ligaments with carbon fibers. Clin Orthop Relat Res 1985;196:169–74.
22. Bercovy M, Goutallier D, Voisin MC, et al. Carbon-PGLA prostheses for ligament reconstruction. Clin Orthop Relat Res 1985;196:159–68.
23. Parsons JR, Bharyani S, Alexander H, et al. Carbon fiber debris within the synovial joint. Clin Orthop Relat Res 1985;196:69–76.
24. Reul GD. Complications in vascular surgery. New York: Grune and Stratton; 1980. p. 631.
25. Magilligan DJ, DeWeese JA. Knot security of synthetic suture materials. Am J Surg 1974;127:355–8.
26. Cooney WP III, Linscheid RL, Dobyns JH. Fractures and dislocations of the wrist. In: Rockwood CA, Green DP, Bucholz RW, editors. Fractures in adults. 3rd edition. Philadelphia: JB Lippincott Company; 1991. p. 563–678.

A Carpal Ligament Substitute Part II

Polyester Suture for Scapho-Lunate and Triqueto-Lunate Ligament Reconstruction

Marwan A. Wehbé, MD[a,b,*], Mary Lee Whitaker, RN[a]

KEYWORDS

- Carpal ligament • Scapholunate • Triquetrolunate • Lunotriquetral • Mersilene • Wrist ligament
- Ligament substitute • Wrist instability

KEY POINTS

- Carpal ligaments are commonly injured and may lead to pain and disability.
- These ligaments are very difficult to repair, and the results are unpredictable.
- A novel approach is presented here using a polyester suture, aiming to substitute these ligaments' function, rather than to repair them.

Carpal ligament function is still a puzzle, in spite of many years of research and advances in the understanding of wrist anatomy and mechanics. Isolated intercarpal ligament ruptures do not seem to lead to gross carpal instability, but they may cause pain and disability. Direct repair of these ligaments does not seem to hold up; witness the numerous supplementary procedures that were developed to reinforce these repairs. Based on the basic observation that the purpose of a ligament is to hold 2 bones in some degree of approximation, the authors propose an alternative method of bone coaptation. The goal of the proposed procedure is to literally tie the 2 involved carpal bones together, such as to restore the function of the interosseous ligament.

DIAGNOSIS

A painful wrist is admittedly difficult to diagnose. A detailed history, physical examination with stress maneuvers, and plain radiographs are a good start. Magnetic resonance imaging (MRI) scan has been disappointing, due to high false-positive and false-negative results. A wrist work-up will usually point to the correct diagnosis, with intraoperative fluoroscopy, arthrogram and arthroscopy. An interosseous ligament tear with no visible instability will respond well to arthroscopic debridement and/or thermal reduction. Large tears usually lead to gross instability and require open treatment for ligament reconstruction.

SURGICAL TECHNIQUE

The procedure is performed while traction is applied to the wrist, using the surgeon's traction apparatus of choice. A bump under the wrist to force the wrist into some flexion during the procedure is also helpful. Fluoroscopy may be used to assist in drill hole placement.

The approach to the wrist depends on which ligament is to be reconstructed. Skin incisions

Disclaimer: Authors have nothing to disclose.
[a] Pennsylvania Hand Center, 101 South Bryn Mawr Avenue, Suite 300, Bryn Mawr, PA 19010, USA; [b] Jefferson Medical College, Philadelphia, PA, USA
* Corresponding author. Pennsylvania Hand Center, 101 South Bryn Mawr Avenue, Suite 300, Bryn Mawr, PA 19010.
E-mail address: Marwan.Wehbé@pahandcenter.com

Hand Clin 29 (2013) 149–154
http://dx.doi.org/10.1016/j.hcl.2012.08.027
0749-0712/13/$ – see front matter © 2013 Elsevier Inc. All rights reserved.

hand.theclinics.com

are laid in a zigzag fashion into the wrist dorsal creases to avoid hypertrophic scars. The approach to the triquetro-lunate (TL) ligament is made through the fifth dorsal compartment.[1] The scapho-lunate (SL) ligament, however, is approached through the fourth dorsal compartment. In the process, the posterior interosseous nerve is identified in the radial aspect of the fourth compartment. A neurectomy of that nerve is performed to help control postoperative pain and, more importantly, to prevent that nerve from getting trapped in the ensuing scar. When both ligaments need to be repaired, the approach will start in the fourth dorsal compartment, and may be extended subcutaneously to the fifth compartment.

The wrist capsule is opened in line with the extrinsic/capsular ligaments. Any ancillary procedures are performed at this time, whether synovectomy or triangular fibrocartilage (TFC) resection. The interosseous ligaments are next visualized. A midsubstance tear is ignored, while a frayed ligament is debrided to prevent it from damaging contiguous cartilage (**Fig. 1A**). A ligament that is avulsed from bone may be repaired, using 1 or 2 bone anchors with nonabsorbable polyester sutures (Micro Quickanchor, with 4-0 Ethibond suture, Dupuy Mitek, Incorporated, Raynham, Massachusetts). There is no evidence that this repair eventually heals or provides any additional strength to the reconstruction.

The main part of the reconstruction involves the coaptation of the bones using 4 strands of polyester 2-0 suture (Mersilene, Johnson & Johnson Ethicon Incorporated, Somerville, New Jersey).[2] A drill hole is made into each of the 2 contiguous bones, from dorsal to palmar in a divergent

fashion, using a 1.5 mm drill bit (see **Fig. 1B** and **Fig. 2**). These holes do not impinge on the articular portion of the carpal bones. The dorsal hole is placed as close to the joint subchondral cortex as possible. The palmar exit hole should be slightly further away from the joint (SL or TL).

A wire suture passer (**Fig. 3**) is inserted into one of the holes and is visualized into the radio-carpal joint (**Fig. 1C**). This wire is retrieved out of the wound with a small single-hook retractor. A 4-0 nylon suture is threaded though the wire passer in the wrist joint and is retrieved dorsally, by pulling the suture passer out. The other end of that nylon suture is passed dorsally with another suture passer, through the other bone (**Fig. 1C**). It is helpful to keep a needle holder on each end of the nylon suture, and a towel clip on the palmar–middle portion of the suture.

Next, a 2-0 Mersilene suture is folded in half, and a simple tie is placed in its middle with one end of the 4-0 nylon (**Fig. 1D**). The nylon suture will be used to thread the Mersilene into the two carpal bones. The towel clip will help pull the nylon with 4 strands of Mersilene into the first hole, then out of the second hole. The nylon is then discarded, and the Mersilene is tied dorsally (**Fig. 1E**). To avoid prominence through skin, the knot is placed over the triquetral tuberosity or dorsal scaphoid ridge. The knot is tied in such a way as to keep it as flat as possible against the carpal bone. The knot may be sewed with 4-0 Mersilene sutures to secure it rather than taking numerous throws, which make it bulky.

By placing the drill holes in a divergent direction from the dorsal approach, the palmar part of the joint closes first while tying the knot (see **Fig. 1E** and

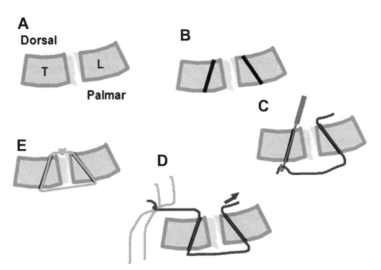

Fig. 1. Diagram showing steps used for Mersilene carpal ligament reconstruction (see text for details). (*Courtesy of* Pennsylvania Hand Center, Bryn Mawr, PA, USA; with permission.)

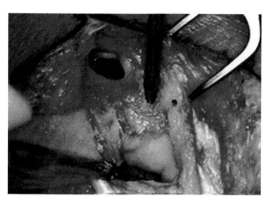

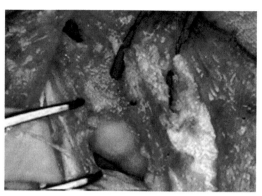

Fig. 2. Intraoperative photograph of a right wrist showing drill bit in lunate. Note the tip of the drill bit in the depth of the wound, at the radio-carpal joint, and the step-off between lunate and triquetrum (*on right side*). The TL ligament is seen avulsed from the lunate. (*Courtesy of* Pennsylvania Hand Center, Bryn Mawr, PA, USA; with permission.)

Fig. 4. Notice how TL space closes while pulling on the Mersilene suture to tie it dorsally. (*Courtesy of* Pennsylvania Hand Center, Bryn Mawr, PA, USA; with permission.)

Fig. 4). This is advantageous, since that part of the joint is in the depth of the wound and cannot be easily visualized. That same Mersilene suture may now be used for the initial closure of the dorsal capsule. More 4-0 Mersilene sutures are used to complete the closure. The extensor retinaculum, which was mostly preserved during the surgical approach, is closed next. There is no need for any Kirschner wire fixation. A bulky bandage and protective splint are applied for edema and pain control.

Following surgery, dressings are changed within 7 to 10 days. Sutures are removed, and a plaster splint or short-arm cast is applied. Protected wrist range of motion (ROM) is not started until 6 weeks after surgery, to allow ample time for fibrous ingrowth into the polyester sutures. Next, a removable wrist cock-up splint is used full-time except for ROM and hygiene for 3 to 4 weeks, then for activity only for another 3 to 4 weeks. All protection is discontinued about 12 weeks postoperatively. Muscle strengthening is started at that time, and unrestricted activities are allowed 4 months after surgery.

HISTOLOGY

Whenever the opportunity arises to visualize a polyester suture that has been implanted for a period of time, the appearance is striking. The sutures are totally incorporated into the scar and ligament remnants (**Fig. 5**).

The histologic appearance of a Mersilene suture 24 months after implantation is shown in **Fig. 6**. This particular specimen came from a 2-0 Mersilene suture that was used for distal radio-ulnar joint (DRUJ) ligament repair, and the ulna head was later resected because of post-traumatic arthrosis (that patient also underwent a TL ligament reconstruction at the time of the DRUJ stabilization). Note the close intertwining of suture material and fibrous tissue. Mersilene polyester sutures have a rough surface, and the polyester weave in essence acts as a scaffolding into which scar tissue is able to grow. Since the polyester is nonabsorbable, the scar tissue ingrowth potentially leads to a construct whose strength increases over time. Although studies were not performed on the properties of Ethibond (Johnson & Johnson Ethicon Incorporated, Somerville, New Jersey), that material's "coating is a relatively nonreactive nonabsorbable compound which

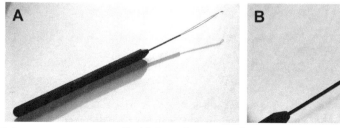

Fig. 3. (*A*) Swanson suture passer (Smith & Nephew, Memphis, Tennessee). (*B*) The tip of the suture passer is bent slightly to facilitate is retrieval with a small hook retractor. (*Courtesy of* Pennsylvania Hand Center, Bryn Mawr, PA, USA; with permission.)

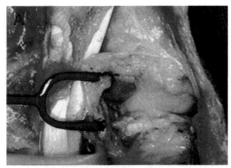
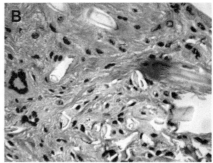

Fig. 5. Findings 24 months after ligament reconstructions with polyester sutures. (*A*) Intraoperative appearance of Mersilene sutures used for TL ligament reconstruction. Wrist joint was explored at time of DRUJ resection. (*B*) Histology of polyester weave suture obtained from dorsal DRU ligament; there is some degree of foreign body reaction, but the polyester fibers are essentially indistinguishable from the surrounding fibrous tissue. (*Courtesy of* Pennsylvania Hand Center, Bryn Mawr, PA, USA; with permission.)

acts as a lubricant"[3] and is likely to prevent this type of ingrowth, since it was designed specifically to prevent tissue adherence.

CLINICAL STUDY

This procedure was performed on 103 wrists since 1985, with follow-up to 15 years. Fifty-five patients with more than 1 year of follow-up were studied retrospectively (range 1–12 years, average 35 months). Forty-eight patients were right-handed, and 7 (13%) were left-handed. Surgery was on the dominant hand in 39 cases (71%), with 5 patients left-handed, and 34 patients right-handed. Sixteen patients (29%) had an SL ligament reconstruction; 35 patients (64%) had TL ligament reconstruction, and 4 patients (7%) had both ligaments reconstructed simultaneously.

Activity level was rated on a scale of 1 to 5 (1 for sedentary, and 5 for heavy labor, such as construction work). The average activity level in this group was 3.19 (range 1–5). Preoperative pain level on a 10-scale ranged between 2 and 6; postoperative pain range was 0 to 5 (**Table 1**). Only 2 patients had pain over 4/10 postoperatively. Fifty-three percent of patients (29 out of the total 55) had complete pain relief within 3 months; the remaining patients were essentially pain-free at final follow-up; those who did have pain described it as related to heavy activity only.

Patients with carpal ligament injuries usually have full ROM, as did all of these patients. Carpal ligament repair does not alter ROM, as long as carpal alignment is maintained. Consequently, ROM remained full in all of these patients. Pain is more of an issue long-term after carpal ligament injuries, and is the result of articular cartilage damage at the time of the initial injury. Witness 2 patients in this group who went on to proximal row carpectomy, and a third who ended up with a wrist fusion.

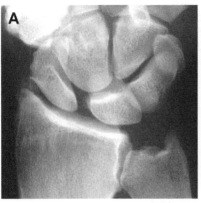
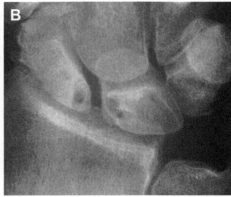

Fig. 6. (*A*) Radiograph showing significant SL gap widening. (*B*) SL gap has been decreased with Mersilene ligament reconstruction. Note the early degenerative changes at the radial styloid and the loose body in that area. A radial styloidectomy may be appropriate in such a case, at the time of ligament reconstruction. (*Courtesy of* Pennsylvania Hand Center, Bryn Mawr, PA, USA; with permission.)

Table 1 Pain levels in 55 patients who underwent Mersilene ligament reconstruction		
Pain Level	**Preoperatively**	**Postoperatively**
0	—	30
1	—	2
2–3	13	17
4–5	35	6
6–7	7	—
8–10	—	—

Grip strength continued to improve up to 1 year after surgery. Predicted grip strength was calculated using the demonstrated assumption that a right hand-dominant person's left hand is 90% of the strength of the right side. A left-handed person, however, has usually equal grip strength in both hands.[4] Preoperative strength was an average of 70% of predicted (range 10% to 100%). Strength at final follow-up was an average of 88% of predicted (range 28% to 112%).

RADIOGRAPHIC APPEARANCE

Radiographic appearance is normal with the majority of carpal ligament injuries. Patients who do have grossly abnormal radiographs, and definitely those with any degenerative changes, do not do well with ligament repairs.

SL ligament deficiency can be corrected with Mersilene ligament reconstruction (**Fig. 6**A). The SL distance can be drastically reduced (**Fig. 6**B), but outcome may be related more to cartilage injury that occurred at the time of injury, or from the intervening period since the injury. One should also keep in mind that correcting SL distance, by itself, may not be enough to correct carpal instability.

The appearance of the drill holes in the carpal bones will vary a great deal, depending on positioning. On rare occasion, the position will be such that a discrete hole is seen in the bone (**Fig. 7**A). More often, however, the bony tunnel will appear as 2 holes or an amorphous shadow (**Fig. 7**B). Making meticulous notes of the gross appearance of the bone tunnels at the time of surgery will alleviate any future concerns about radiographic appearance.

DISCUSSION

Carpal ligament injuries have been described extensively.[5] Interosseous (intrinsic) ligament tears are quite common, but are not easily diagnosed without simultaneous capsular injury leading to gross instability. Standard radiographs, even with dynamic and stress views, may appear normal, and advanced imaging (computed tomography [CT] and MRI) is not likely to be contributory either.[6] Even without carpal instability and normal radiographic appearance, however, a torn carpal ligament can be a source of pain.[7] The diagnosis is often made surgically, with a wrist work-up consisting of intraoperative fluoroscopy, arthrograms, and arthroscopy.[8,9]

The major intrinsic ligaments are the SL and TL ligaments. These ligaments have a membranous central (proximal) portion, and are ligamentous in their dorsal and palmar portions. A tear in the membranous portion will not produce any instability, but may be a source of pain and post-traumatic arthrosis.[10,11]

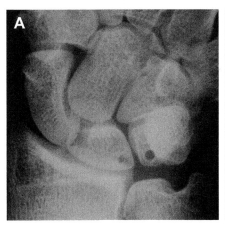 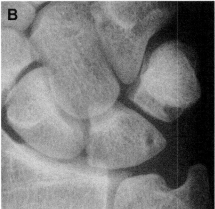

Fig. 7. Radiographic appearance of a wrist after TL ligament reconstruction. (*A*) Wrist is in ulnar deviation, and hole in triquetrum happens to be facing the x-ray beam. (*B*) Wrist is in radial deviation, and neither drill hole looks like a bony tunnel. (*Courtesy of* Pennsylvania Hand Center, Bryn Mawr, PA, USA; with permission.)

Various procedures have been devised to make up for the structural deficits that follow carpal ligament injuries.[12,13] These consist of various forms of capsulodesis or tenodesis, or combinations thereof, rather than direct ligament repair. Tendons used to replace ligaments cannot fare well; these tendons have not been proven to survive as structurally potent structures, and may not be able to absorb the loads applied to wrist ligaments. There are also proponents of carpal fusions, which totally bypass the issue of ligament reconstruction.[14–18]

The SL ligament is among the strongest ligaments in the human body. Its strength has been determined to be around 359 N.[19] We have determined that 4 strands of Mersilene polyester suture actually exceed 400 N.[20] The property demonstrated by this uncoated polyester suture to invite fibrous ingrowth could even lead to a stronger construct over time. Stress testing of embedded polyester sutures in vivo has not, however, been performed. The procedure described here places the ligament reconstruction dorsally and palmar, thus restoring ligament strength where it is normally needed.[21]

The failure of ligament reconstructions in this series was found to be due, primarily, to cartilage injury and post-traumatic arthrosis, rather than to failure of the ligament repair. A decision needs to be made for each case whether a ligament reconstruction should be attempted, or whether one should resort to a salvage procedure from the outset.[22]

Mersilene polyester sutures have the strength needed to repair or substitute for ligaments in vivo. They may be used for the reconstruction of carpal ligaments, and they should also be considered for ligament repair elsewhere.

REFERENCES

1. Wehbé MA. Surgical approach to the ulnar wrist. J Hand Surg 1986;11A:509–12.
2. Available at: http://www.ecatalog.ethicon.com/sutures-non-absorbable/view/mersilene-suture. Accessed October 1, 2012.
3. Available at: http://www.ecatalog.ethicon.com/sutures-non-absorbable/view/ethibond-excel-suture. Accessed October 1, 2012.
4. Crosby CA, Wehbé MA. Hand strength normative values. J Hand Surg 1994;19A:665–70.
5. Linscheid RL, Dobyns JH, Beabout JW, et al. Traumatic instability of the wrist—diagnosis, classification, and pathomechanics. J Bone Joint Surg Am 1972;54A:1612–32.
6. Cautilli GP, Wehbé MA. Scapho-lunate distance and cortical ring sign. J Hand Surg 1991;16A:501–3.
7. Taleisnik J. The ligaments of the wrist. J Hand Surg 1976;1:110.
8. Profas JM, Jackson WT. Evaluating carpal instabilities with fluoroscopy. AJR Am J Roentgenol 1980;135:137–40.
9. Wehbé MA, Parisien JS. Arthroscopy of the wrist. In: Parisien JS, editor. Arthroscopic surgery, volume 24. New York: McGraw-Hill; 1987. p. 293–9.
10. Green DP. Operative hand surgery. 2nd edition. New York: Churchill Livingstone; 1988. p. 917.
11. Ruby LK, Stinson J, Belsky M. The natural history of scaphoid non-union. J Bone Joint Surg Am 1985;67:428–32.
12. Lavernia CJ, Cohen MS, Taleisnik J. Treatment of scapholunate dissociation by ligamentous repair and capsulodesis. J Hand Surg Am 1992;17:354–9.
13. Lichtman DM, Bruckner JD, Culp RW, et al. Palmar midcarpal instability: results of surgical reconstruction. J Hand Surg 1993;18A:307–15.
14. Minami A, Ogino T, Minami M. Limited wrist fusions. J Hand Surg 1988;13A:660–7.
15. Trumble T, Bour CJ, Smith RJ, et al. Intercarpal arthrodesis for static and dynamic volar intercalated segment instability. J Hand Surg 1988;13A:384–91.
16. Watson HK, Vender M. Wrist and intercarpal arthrodesis. In: Chapman M, editor. Operative orthopedics. 2nd edition. Philadelphia: Lippincott; 1993. p. 1363.
17. Wehbé MA, Dick HD, Beckenbaugh RD, et al. Salvage options after wrist trauma: alternatives to fusion. Presented at the Symposium of the American Society for Surgery of the Hand. Orlando, Florida, October 4, 1994.
18. Augsburger S, Necking L, Horton J, et al. A comparison of scaphoid-trapezium-trapezoid fusion and four-bone tendon weave for scapholunate dissociation. J Hand Surg 1992;17A:360–9.
19. Mayfied JK, Williams WJ. Biomechanical properties of human carpal ligaments. Orthop Transactions 1979;3:143–4.
20. Martin JA, Wehbé MA. A carpal ligament substitute: part 1. Polyester suture. Hand Clinics 2013.
21. Berger RA, Toshihiko I, Berglund L, et al. Constraint and material properties of the subregions of the scapho-lunate interosseous ligament. J Hand Surg 1999;24A:953–62.
22. Palmer AK, Dobyns JH, Linscheid RL. Management of post-traumatic instability of the wrist secondary to ligament rupture. J Hand Surg 1978;3:507–32.

Index

Note: Page numbers of article titles are in **boldface** type.

A

Artelon, in trapezium prosthetic arthroplasty, 40–41

Arthroplasty, around wrist, history and design considerations for, **1–13**
  general postoperative care following, 124

Avanta prosthesis, for trapezium prosthetic arthroplasty, 46, 47

B

Basal arthritis, of thumb, ligament reconstruction and tendon interposition for, **15–25**

Biaxial total wrist, 5

Braun-Cutter prosthesis, for trapezium prosthetic arthroplasty, 44, 45

C

Carpal collapse, scaphotrapezial-trapezoid fusion in, 2

Carpal ligament, function of, diagnosis of, 149

Carpal ligament substitute, polyester suture as, **143–148**
  clinical study of, 152–153
  discussion of, 147, 153–154
  for scapho- and triqueto-ligament reconstruction, **149–154**
  histology of, 151–152
  radiographic appearance of, 152, 153
  surgical technique for, 149–151

Carpectomy, proximal row, **69–78**
  alternative techniques for, 76–77
  description of, 69
  in acute injury, 74–75
  in chronic perilunate injury, 74
  in Kienbock's disease, 74
  indications for, 70
  operative technique for, 70–72
  outcomes of, 73–75
  postoperative care following, 72–73
  postoperative evaluation in, 73
  preoperative evaluation for, 70
  wrist arthrodesis and, 75–76

Carpometacarpal joint(s). See also *Thumb, carpometacarpal joint of.*
  and scaphoid-trapezium joint arthroplasty, **57–68**
  II and III, arthroplasty of, 61–63
    carpal bossing and, 61–62, 63

complications of, 63
  resection arthroplasty of, 62–63
IV and V, arthroplasty of, 63–66
  complications of, 66
  partial resection arthroplasty of, 65
  resection arthroplasty of, with arthrodesis, 65–66
  simple implant arthroplasty of, 64
  tendon interposition arthroplasty of, 65

Cooney prosthesis, for trapezium prosthetic arthroplasty, 45–46

Cottony Dacron, as carpal ligament substitute, 143–145

D

Darrach and Sauvé-Kapandji procedure, clinical outcomes of, 104

de la Caffinière prosthesis, for trapezium prosthetic arthroplasty, 41–42

Derotation sling, 139, 140

E

Elektra prosthesis, for trapezium prosthetic arthroplasty, 42–44

Ethibond, as carpal ligament substitute, 143–145, 146, 147

Exercises, range of motion, following arthroplasty, 124
  tendon gliding, following arthroplasty, 124

Extensor pollicis brevis, transfer of, in management of basal arthritis of thumb, 22, 23

F

Flexor carpi radialis harvest, in management of basal arthritis of thumb, 18–19, 20

Forearm, rotation of, measurements of, following arthroplasty, 125–126, 127
  radioulnar joints and, 103–104

Fractures, of wrist, periprosthetic management of, 9

G

Gonimeter, to measure forearm rotation, 126, 127
  to measure wrist extention, 125

http://dx.doi.org/10.1016/S0749-0712(12)00150-3
0749-0712/13/$ – see front matter © 2013 Elsevier Inc. All rights reserved.

Moving?

Make sure your subscription moves with you!

To notify us of your new address, find your **Clinics Account Number** (located on your mailing label above your name), and contact customer service at:

Email: journalscustomerservice-usa@elsevier.com

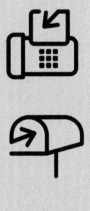

800-654-2452 (subscribers in the U.S. & Canada)
314-447-8871 (subscribers outside of the U.S. & Canada)

Fax number: 314-447-8029

Elsevier Health Sciences Division
Subscription Customer Service
3251 Riverport Lane
Maryland Heights, MO 63043

*To ensure uninterrupted delivery of your subscription, please notify us at least 4 weeks in advance of move.

Printed and bound by CPI Group (UK) Ltd, Croydon, CR0 4YY

03/10/2024

01040346-0016

.